Reader Comments

Terry Shouba has given us a wise, moving, and beautifully written account of what it is really like to be "in therapy." This is a valuable resource for anyone contemplating getting psychotherapeutic help, and especially so for those, like so many of our soldiers and former soldiers, who are hesitating because of the stigma associated with emotional suffering. Her book takes the mystery out a healing process that can relieve much pain, and at times be life-saving.

—Neal Spira, MD, President Chicago Psychoanalytic Society,
Associate Dean Chicago Institute for Psychoanalysis

A wise, perceptive, sympathetic book.

—MDH

It's like becoming a whole new person, this process...I suppose you're just getting introduced to parts of yourself you didn't know very well, but it feels like those parts are being born anew. Either way, it's exciting and scary and tremendously hard and also very joyful, at times.

—HCT

Conversations About Therapy is an eye-opening work written by one who has spent her time in the trenches of life. It offers an unvarnished look at the stigma of mental health issues and professional therapy/counseling. Gently but honestly giving voice to "everyday people", Terry Shouba is an important part of the "cadre of determined people beating back stigma surrounding emotional problems." As a pastor, I appreciate the healing pathway she is creating for others, as well as her creative writing offered with deep insight and heartfelt compassion.

—Rev. Steven Good

It would certainly encourage people who are struggling in therapy to keep going. I know that it would have helped me when I was in therapy to have realized other people were having the same issues as me. Sometimes, in the early days, I used to think that the thoughts I had about therapy, but didn't always share with my therapist, were just me being crazy. Now I know others have the same thoughts.

—LWF

The clients' comments, and your own, are enlightening to a therapist or therapist-to-be, and many times represent issues that are not discussed in full in each person's therapy.

—Kathy Hotelling, PhD, ABPP

I am in awe of your strength not to commit suicide—I'm inspired by your example of moving on to a fuller, happier life, and I applaud your courage to openly share your story so that others might also come to know a more joyful existence.

BE

AF798648

This a terrific book which I would readily recommend to anyone who is considering psychotherapy or embarking on it. The author clearly describes all the elements of the therapy process with sophistication and compassion, leaving jargon behind as she weaves together experiences and stories of real people in treatment. With considerable depth, she clarifies a complex process that nevertheless appreciates that being in therapy isn't simple and that it is always ultimately unique for each patient as well as for each patient/therapist relationship.

I would have found this book incredibly useful when, well before I was a psychologist, I looked for books in order to hear the voices of people like me, or with whom I could identify, describe their stories of distress and repair, and something more about the process from the patient's point of view. There were not many such books around. This book would have been of great help—and will be now for others—as it wonderfully gives voice and context to the process of psychotherapy.

—Dale Young, PsyD, psychologist in private practice, Boston;
Co-author, *The Complete Guide to Mental Health for Women*;
Advanced Candidate, Boston Institute for Psychoanalysis

It's a sad and daunting process, for sure. But I feel really confident that I'll be a happier, healthier person when it's over. I haven't been very honest with myself for a lot of years and now that I'm tapping in to what I've truly been feeling, it's liberating in all kinds of unexpected ways. Even when the feelings are sad, it's just refreshing to let myself feel them...And my newfound therapist (found after reading your book!!) is an absolute lifeline.

—RKG

Conversations About Therapy supports and encourages all who are curious about beginning the path to emotional well-being and self-discovery. Through the sharing of personal experiences, her own and those she interviewed, Terryl Shouba brings perspective to a relationship that's not often discussed: client and therapist. She explores the challenges that confront those who consider, and also who follow through with, the therapeutic process. She asks the questions that many of us, familiar or not with therapy, would like to have answered. The book is an immensely useful tool and a behind-the-scenes look at what is involved when beginning and continuing in therapy.

—AD

I don't think anyone has written a book like this that shows the perspective of the people in therapy...The stories are fascinating and humbling. Each story is different and yet there are common threads that run through each of them.

—SIK

CONVERSATIONS ABOUT THERAPY

PEOPLE TELL THEIR STORIES

TERRYL KINNEAR SHOUBA

MARSH HOUSE BOOKS

St. Charles, Illinois

2013

MARSH HOUSE BOOKS

St. Charles, Illinois

Copyright © 2013 by Terryl Kinnear Shouba

ISBN 978-0-578-11054-7

Library of Congress Catalog number: 2012915345

All rights reserved. No part of this publication may be reproduced, stored in a retrieval system or transmitted, in any form, or by any means, electronic, mechanical, recorded, photocopied, or otherwise, without the prior written permission of both the copyright owner and the above publisher of this book, except by a reviewer who may quote brief passages in a review.

The scanning, uploading, and distribution of this book via the Internet or via any other means without the permission of the publisher is illegal and punishable by law. Please purchase only authorized electronic editions and do not participate in or encourage electronic piracy of copyrightable materials. Your support of the author's rights is appreciated.

Printed in the United States of America

Contents

With gratitude to Michael Hoit, M.D.
—psychoanalyst, conjuror,
mother, father, healer, friend—
who stayed steady in the boat
and never gave up on me

The most exciting journey you will ever take
is the one to your own mind.

–therapist of Mary O, artist

Give sorrow words. The grief that does not speak
Whispers the o'er-fraught heart and bids it break.

- William Shakespeare,
Macbeth, Act IV, Scene 3

Only injuries thoroughly cleaned can heal.

–Michelle Bachelet,
in dedicating the Museum of Memory
and Human Rights
Santiago, Chile

Foreword

IF you ever thought about seeking help for your emotional problems, whether they stem from your troubled past, your relationship with loved ones or peers, or the adversities that life presents you, you might have hesitated because of the many questions that you had. You might have asked yourself, "How do I decide if I need or do not need to do this? Who could I trust enough with the details of my private life and deepest thoughts? Where would I find such a person? What would it be like to sit and talk with a stranger about such personal matters? What could such a person say that would possibly help or make a difference? How will I deal with the issue of revealing to others that I am engaged in such a task? Will it affect my relationship with those with whom I am involved for the better or for the worse?" Lastly, "Perhaps I am better off doing nothing and handling matters myself no matter the consequences! Maybe it will all go away!"

If you ever had such thoughts or questions, this book might help you decide what course of action to take. Here you will find the stories, collected by Terry and sensitively rendered, of twelve people from varied backgrounds with diverse problems talking about their experiences in the process we call "psychotherapy." I once had a patient who asked me "What is 'psycho' therapy?" I detected his skepticism and distrust of any involvement, and took note of the disparagement implied by his thinking it was something more appropriate for "psychos."

I tried to be reassuring by saying that it simply was a form of counseling. Counseling seemed to him to be a much friendlier term to describe the process involved in talking with someone about one's troubles. After all, the function of counselor has a centuries-long tradition among those we call pastors and priests. They are people who have devoted their lives to serving God and helping others. What is different about psychotherapists is that they come from a profession that has its origins in a more recent invention. They are part of a trend that seeks to professionalize the discipline by placing it on a scientific foundation, such as exists in the medical profession.

There are three major professions that provide psychotherapy services: psychiatrists, clinical psychologists, and clinical social workers. The differences among them are that psychiatrists can prescribe medications, whereas the other two cannot; clinical psychologists may at times administer psychological tests to collect information about the person's functioning; clinical social workers, in addition to their work on psychological issues, will have an interest in helping people with problems related to their environment. The common element among them is that almost all of them use talk therapy to improve people's conditions. They often come from different theoretical orientations, which means that each individual therapist may use different techniques in how they work with people.

In this highly informative book, Terry has organized the materials she collected from her interviews along some helpful headings that serve as guides for the reader. She provides details of what drove some to seek help, how they went about finding someone to talk to, what it was like to be involved in such a process, how it helped and impacted their lives.

In reading about these people's experiences, you may see yourselves and may be encouraged to consider whether such a step might be right for you. It is not a decision to be made lightly, but if you do make it and you in fact find a psychotherapist with whom you are able to make a connection, you will later on find that the decision was among the most worthwhile ones that you have made in your life.

Joseph Palombo
Founding Dean
Institute for Clinical Social Work, Chicago

Dear Reader—

Therapy is a scary prospect, as all of these stories illustrate. Even reading about it can be unsettling. But I believe that learning about others' experiences in therapy helps us to think about our own.

You might think therapy is just for other people. Or that seeing a therapist signals something peculiar about you. I was convinced for years that I was somehow different from other people until I talked to the men and women in this book—and saw how much we had in common. Though it was therapy that changed me, their stories helped to change how I felt about therapy. Instead of shame, I very slowly began to see not just what was "wrong" with me, but also my courage and persistence; imagine that.

This is also true: "there is no bright line separating health from illness, distress from disease." The voices in this book belong to everyday people with the same kinds of problems as people you know. Their unexpected, touching, wise, and funny comments gave me a new perspective. Maybe they will do that for you.

Some books are sacred texts that can't be marked or underlined. But this is a book of conversations and I invite you to be part of them. Feel free to underline and write your own comments in the margins. Add the date. Make the book yours. These notes become benchmarks of your growth. Each time you read certain passages you will discover something new, and that is growth happening in tiny increments. This happened to me repeatedly during the years I pored over the transcript of others' thoughts and feelings, trying to figure out how to respond. Bewildered, I would ask myself, "How could I have missed that?" I would find new meaning in something that had slipped past me many, many times.

The process of deciding on therapy can be overwhelming. Maybe one day you'll say, "I need to let someone help me." Or maybe you think, "I could never talk about that." But you might be surprised by what you can talk about with someone you grow to trust who cares about you, without judgment. And astonished by what enormous relief it brings. Maybe one day you will think about this book and say, "Now I get it—I didn't before, but now I do."

Books can change lives. This one might help you find the courage to change yours.

—TS

PART ONE

The Man in the Waiting Room

> You can out-distance that which is running after you, but not what is running inside you.
>
> Rwandan Proverb

MAPLE trees glowed in the morning light as I drove to my appointment, arriving in the waiting room of my therapist's office with a few minutes to spare. A man, sitting quietly, didn't look at me. Taking the ladies room key from the hook, I stepped out to the hall. When I returned I saw my doctor shake the man's hand, heard the man say he was early, then heard the doctor's reassuring voice reply that he would see him next.

When the office door closed behind me, I hesitated, then mentioned that the man appeared to be in such pain. It was none of my business. I didn't say so, but it almost hurt to look at him. He wore sunglasses, which I used to do when my eyes were red from crying or I was trying to hide. He smelled of alcohol and his body, clutching a black canvas portfolio, was almost contorted in tension. I wondered how long he had taken to ask for help and hoped he would not give up.

Then, as we had done so many times in that quiet space, we began to talk. Yet the memory of the man in the waiting room stayed with me long after my appointment ended.

What is the book about?

Imagine a place where you could talk about anything at all, knowing it would be held in confidence, without fear of being cast out; someplace safe. Imagine making sense of all the puzzling pieces of your emotional life, draining your anger, thinning out your sorrows, then returning to the world more confident and self-aware, no longer feeling different from others or oddly furtive. Imagine a place where you could learn to trust again, to give and receive love, and to live with yourself. Imagine: a therapist's office.

Despite the prospect of emotional peace, many of us shun the idea of therapy or avoid taking steps to get ourselves in the actual chair. Beyond the problems of cost and access to quality mental health care loom further obstacles. The fear of what others would think, if they knew, is fueled by sketchy ideas of what therapy is—or could be. Except for an improbable mention to close confidants, none of us talks about our therapy. Mostly we don't ask and don't tell. Our collective silence compounds misconceptions about what therapy is and what it can accomplish.

These are among the topics of these conversations about therapy, where people who refused to accept the status quo agreed to talk about their experiences in therapy: how we got there, why we stay (or leave), and changes therapy brought about.

Who is the book written for?

This book is written for individuals who are contemplating therapy and their loved ones. We know little about other people's experiences in therapy. I learned from the interviews that unrealistic expectations abound, and that therapy's countless benefits are kept rather private. It needs to be more widely known how much relief the perspective of a caring, listening person can bring—and with it, the courage to rebuild in the face of loss.

Those of us who are weighed down by emotional problems soon learn that we alone bear responsibility to understand ourselves and change. No one else can save us. We can remain stuck with our problems, trying every remedy on earth to avoid facing ourselves, or we can undertake a journey of learning and self-discovery. If we set out on a path of self-knowledge, aided by an able therapist, we can be sure of the uncertainty of its length and of what we will find. What is certain is that the way, though difficult, will make an important difference in our lives; under certain conditions, even a profound difference.

Why does it matter?

Setting anecdotal evidence and intuition aside for a moment, data in this matter are compelling. In terms of disability, the burden of major depression is equal to blindness or paraplegia. Mental disorders affect one of every five Americans; worldwide, they are slightly more prevalent than all forms of cancer combined. Here is another important fact: of the top thirteen non-contagious diseases—this includes cancer and heart disease—*neuropsychiatric conditions are the leading cause of death.*[1] Data such as these, analyzed for a study conducted on a worldwide scale by the World Health Organization, the World Bank, and the Harvard School of Public Health, present a somber picture of psychiatric disorders in a context of other illness and disease.

> NIMH **Global Cost of Mental Illness**
>
> ...the global cost of mental illness at nearly $2.5T (two-thirds in indirect costs) in 2010, with a projected increase to over $6T by 2030. What does $2.5T or $6T mean? The entire global health spending in 2009 was $5.1T. The annual GDP for low-income countries is less than $1T. The entire overseas development aid over the past 20 years is less than $2T.[2]

Despite the prevalence of emotional burdens in all forms and sizes, the shame of having "problems" keeps many people from seeking help even if they can afford it. We don't know much about the whole business, the prospect is scary, and what happens in the therapeutic space is a mystery to most of us. Why do people go? Why do some find it so helpful and others reject it? Why do people suffer with unnecessary pain, settle into disappointing relationships, or end their lives rather than go into therapy and stay until the job is done? These questions are worth asking because the cost of unattended emotional disorder—in terms of personal suffering, premature death, family unhappiness, illness, and crime—is staggering.

Medical professionals, with the obvious exception of psychiatrists, tend to evaluate physical symptoms through a lens of the systems and processes of the human body, giving scant attention to the possibility that some physical conditions, even many, may have an emotional origin, albeit one that is deeply buried, which is what happens with trauma. Take an apparently healthy young person who dies inexplicably at the same age as a beloved parent, as if the impact of such profound loss had been lodged inside the heart, with fatal implications.

Shrouded in whispers and misconceptions, therapy needs to become as accepted and commonplace as breakfast cereal. This is not to reveal personal issues, but rather so that those who embrace it will become more open about it, sharing why they go into therapy and what happens there. Many people give up on themselves, ashamed of their failure to thrive, unaware of the degree to which others, usually in strict privacy, use therapy to unburden themselves, strengthen their vitality, and redirect their lives. Therapists know this, but many who wander lost in their own lives may not.

Emotional problems are largely a matter of degree. No line is drawn between those who have them and those who don't. They afflict the rich, famous, and well educated as well as the rest of us. The term "mental illness" is hazy and stigmatizing. No one wants to stand under its black umbrella. Yet still the term is used to label people, as if emotional problems alone could define any of us.

In some people's minds, all mental problems are lumped together, helping them believe they are exempt, even superior. Sometimes those who are most opposed to therapy, even most inclined to denounce it or most contemptuous of it, are the ones who are least aware of a part of themselves they don't want to know.

The following portraits of people's experiences in therapy show how it helped them achieve greater self-knowledge, a sturdier foundation of confidence, and more compassion. You may not agree with some of the interviewees' comments, but what they say is instructive.

Interspersed among the "conversations" are excerpts from research publications of the National Institute for Mental Health. Despite the ill-chosen term "mental illness," the excerpts underscore the fact that for many of us the seeds of emotional problems are sown early and that these disorders, or symptoms, specified as this or that "mental illness"—panic disorder or obsessive-compulsive disorder, or whatever disorder—spill not only into each other, but also into our physical well-being, as if it is all one and the same; which it is. So the NIMH excerpts are a backdrop to the stories, suggesting the scope of such problems on a larger stage, far greater than our dozen voices.

NIMH Mental Illness and Other Illnesses

Mental illness alone will account for more than half of the projected total economic burden from [non-communicable diseases] over the next two decades and 35% of the global lost output. Considering that those with mental illness are at high risk for developing cardiovascular disease, respiratory disease, and diabetes, the true costs of mental illness must be even higher.[3]

When therapy emerges from the shadows, its many dimensions are shown in a warmer light. With greater awareness of mental health in our society, we can no longer lump everything under "mental illness." Many lives are enriched with short-term interventions. For others of us, it goes far beyond that: it is the only chance we have to save ourselves, the only chance to have any kind of life.

How did the idea for the book originate?

The idea emerged when several strands in my life came together like streams to a river. I had recently left a job teaching a middle-school classroom of students with emotional and behavior disorders, giving me more time to read and think. Among my circle of friends I learned that two were shut out and stigmatized for issues related to mental health. One was denied health insurance because he took antidepressants and another was denied a job with the Federal government because in college she had been briefly in therapy following the sudden death of her father, as if this were a felony. The third strand was my growing awareness of the many people who don't seek help.

Another strand was finding a new book by Robert Coles, M.D. A child psychiatrist, he had captured in many of his books the voices of children who were trying to make sense of circumstances of their lives in families of migrant workers, in war-torn countries, or amid racial violence. Of those I had read, I noticed how closely and respectfully he listened to what each child had to say. To him, their thoughts and ideas mattered. His new book was *Lives of Moral Leadership*, in the voices of adults, some famous and others not. I read it and decided (tentatively at first) that I would find a way to write about the one thing I knew something about.

Maybe it was around this time that I saw the man in the waiting room, and he was the catalyst. I do remember driving home from one of my appointments when the idea for this book came to me, pulling over to the side of the road to write down interview questions as they arrived in one uninterrupted stream.

The idea offered an intriguing opportunity to explore some issues related to therapy. I wondered why I had stayed in therapy while others left, resigning themselves to conditions in their lives that I felt, albeit as an outsider, would not be necessary if they continued in treatment. If I had changed, why couldn't they? Those who were considering therapy from any vantage point might be interested to learn how and why others made certain decisions along the way.

As I found people to interview and began writing, I came to see stigma as a schoolyard bully. Stigma, with its mighty irrational power, intimidates us and keeps us from listening to messages from our own hearts. I felt this book could stand up to stigma, strip it of some of its power, and stare it down.

The idea for the book was simple enough. Through interviews, readers would hear the voices of men and women who had gone into therapy—those who had resolved the issues that drew them into treatment, and those who continued, sometimes for many years, to work with a therapist. It would foster acceptance of how relative is therapy's time and pace, how infinite yet dimly knowable are the reaches of our minds. If just a few people shared their experiences of therapy, others might see that for some of us the experience was not just useful but life-saving and life-enriching, possibilities previously beyond our imagining.

How did the book come into being?

The book also began with a woman I'll call Sarah. Like everyone I interviewed, her name has been changed. We met when I was a training consultant at a company where she worked. After the assignment ended we began to see each other less often. Then one day she called to say she wanted to get together at my house rather than in a café, where we usually met. She settled into our old blue sofa looking happy and pretty, but a little uneasy. She told me that she and her husband were separating, that he had a drinking problem he wouldn't deal with, that she had met someone else. The story tumbled out of her.

As I listened, I remember gazing through the window at the dappled light in the trees and realizing how painful it is to listen to other people's problems.

I also saw how much she needed to be listened to, heard, and accepted, and how much relief she felt when it happened—I could see it in her face.

At the time I felt, and perhaps this is another strand, that even though I am not a therapist, my years in therapy could modestly qualify me to be an interviewer, observer, and recorder of others' experiences. Our perspective as clients, or patients, is from *inside* the experience of therapy. Here the battles are fought; here the insights and changes take place. It is from here, where we make ourselves vulnerable, that we find our way out of torment—if we are willing to commit to the process.

So, angry and curious about the stigma of being in therapy—for myself, my friends, my former students, others I read about or had known over the years—I called Sarah. She embraced the idea and was the first person to be interviewed. As the "playwright" I wanted to have a main character on which to hang the so-called plot, so I chose Sarah's story to open each chapter, though hers is no more important than others. Also, despite limited financial resources, she never gave up. I found her fortitude inspiring.

Another source of inspiration was a song I happened to hear, "Dear Someone," by Gillian Welch. It gave me the idea of a way to address a letter to prospective interview candidates that could be placed on an information table at churches, temples, college counseling centers. I met with several members of the clergy to describe the project and ask if they would make my letter available. Only I would know if anyone responded. The early encouragement of a few of these individuals meant a great deal to me. Everyone I interviewed came because of the letter, a referral, or my direct request.

I was also encouraged from another unexpected source. In the early months of my effort, as I reached out to find people to interview—I didn't want any of my participants to know any of the others—a minister referred me to a therapist who agreed to talk with me. At the end of our meeting he held up a book, suggesting I call its author. The cover read *Learning Disorders and Disorders of the Self in Children and Adolescents* by Joseph Palombo. Mr. Palombo, a distinguished therapist in Chicago, works with people who have learning disabilities, understanding them from clinical and neuroscience perspectives. As a former teacher, I was intrigued by the title. So I called him, explaining the book I wanted to write, and he said, "I'm very interested in your idea."

We met not long afterward—only once, but I took careful notes. As the months went on (and on), I sent each sprawling chapter to Joe, who would e-mail encouragement. Without his caring and gentle support, his years of faith in me and this book, the idea would have remained only that. Because of him and those who share their stories, this is our book, not just mine. In that spirit, a portion of the proceeds from the sale of this book are being donated to the Institute for Clinical Social Work to be used in treating individuals whose access to care is limited.

And so, the project was like embarking on a voyage to some unknown land in a seaworthy little boat, buoyed by the reassurances of experienced sailors (Joe and my therapist) that this idea had merit.

How is the book organized?

The background in Part One sets the stage for the conversations about therapy that follow; it also includes my story. Part Two consists of interview excerpts in chapters organized around specific topics: how we came to decide on therapy, found a therapist, thought about the experience and its meaning in our lives, and wrestled with issues of medication (or not), finances, insurance (or not), the reactions of family and friends to our endeavor, and the decision to end therapy (or not). Part Three offers concluding thoughts.

During the interviews I tried not to intrude on anyone's train of thought. In my selection of excerpts from each transcript, I highlighted those that felt important. Everything is filtered through a prism of my experience in the care of a very good therapist over a period of many years.

The book's straightforward format and its loose parallel to the therapeutic process give a structure for thinking about therapy. We see issues that many people have in common, such as their fears about therapy, problems finding a therapist, and ways of gauging progress. Those who need it may feel encouraged to keep trying: to find a good therapist, to keep working at it, and not to expect too much, too soon. I tried to replicate the back-and-forth quality of a conversation in therapy: an individual's response to a question followed by my reflection as a fellow patient. Although I offer some conclusions, they are mostly left to you, the reader, because the choice of a therapist is highly individual as is the judgment of what does and doesn't work.

To help my participants feel more at ease, I said that I would also tell my story. That has proved harder to do than I had at first thought, but it has helped me understand how hard it must have been for them. It reminded me how important it is that one's therapist has also sat in the other chair and knows just how difficult it can be.

MY STORY

Thousands of books tell the sad stories of troubled families whose children bear the traces in their souls. These are often stories about overcoming adversity. One puzzling feature—I have read a good many of them—is that therapy is glossed over. As one woman vaguely put it, "I needed time to sort through old burdens." In all of them I wanted to ask, "How did you come to terms with what happened? How did you overcome the shame—or did you? Was all that time and money worth it?" I wanted to ask, "Where are the stories of those whose courage and persistence in therapy brought them a different, private triumph? Where are stories, as viewed from the inside, of people whose lives were made better because of therapy?"

Shortly after beginning to see a new therapist ("H.") I asked him outright if he knew the way out of the cave of hopelessness to which I kept returning. Yes, he nodded. And he did, though I wanted to give up on him, on therapy, and on myself many, many times. The work was hard and the rewards, for a long time, were barely noticeable. I kept losing heart and could not see the changes slowly forming, but he must have. Meanwhile everyone else's life—I was sure of it—hummed along while mine was mired in the muck of depression, anxiety, and assorted other psychic afflictions.

I had begun to see H. as a new divorcee with two young children, arriving in Chicago one bitter January as my one year of alimony expired. Another psychoanalyst had recommended him. My choice was based on the only satisfactory experience in therapy I'd had after a series of failed efforts with various other therapists to right myself, like a boat whose sail drags in the water. Although there are stories far worse than mine, I can see now how much destruction took place in the years I lived in my family, taking a darker turn the summer I was sixteen.

That summer my severely depressed mother was confined to a psychiatric hospital. She was allowed no visitors that first month. In the next month our few visits were brief. At home I tried to cook and keep house for my father and me. One late August night he surprised us both by trying to seduce me. That's all it was. The details aren't pertinent here, but like a ball that falls outside a boundary, he had crossed the incest line, silently detonating a sacred trust. Something within me broke, registering in my body, but beyond reach of my conscious mind. We never spoke of it, as if it never happened.

In pictures of myself in the first years afterward, I see the face of someone who was hardly there. For perhaps a few decades I don't recall ever thinking about what happened, maybe trying to cordon it off to a part of my mind saved for things that can't be reckoned with at the time. I couldn't see that it was anything except some words, and how could they be anything? I couldn't see that the center of myself wouldn't hold together.

Within the first year of seeing H., I must have mentioned the August night with my father. He knew early on, but we didn't talk about it again for many years, and then possibly only in little bits. Maybe he waited until I was ready. For years, every attempt to speak of it ended in overwhelming terror. We began, sometimes with intervening years, the arduous work of finding pieces that had fallen out of the picture, which is to say all of them.

We began to talk, because the evidence appeared in every session and in every day of my life, about how it had felt to have my father call me stupid, to realize how much pleasure it gave him to inflict pain on me, to return to the memories of his knuckle digging into my back, twisting my fingers, mocking me, calling me names, showering me with expletives from an anger he couldn't contain. I hear my mother's voice, "Stop it! Stop hurting her!" and he laughs, disgusted with my tears. I hear his voice, ordering, then, "or I'll knock your block off." Even so, I adored him. Remembrance in undertaking such unearthly work is painstakingly slow.

I didn't know—no one did—the connection between any of this and the altered teenager who waited for the morning school bus. My mother returned home from the hospital, pale and thin. No one spoke of her time away. Our days resumed like a quiet clock, but somewhere in my mind a trap door opened and I had fallen through it. Even if I had known what happened, I could never have told her, knowing I would be blamed, as I felt I deserved to be.

One day out of the blue my high school counselor asked my parents to meet with her. That had never happened before. I had been a model student. The same counselor had reassured me that I was intelligent enough to go to college. I asked her because I wasn't sure, having been reminded so often of my stupidity. They met while I sang in the choir at a school assembly. Somehow the honors student had vanished and in her place was someone failing her classes, truant from school, and with her fingernails scraping her arms till they bled. I had no memory of what had or hadn't happened, no idea that my father, as I had known him, could no longer be my father, nor that the gulf between my fragile mother and me would widen further. After the meeting I was sent to a psychiatrist three times a week and went to school half days until, after careful tending, I left for college.

Not until decades later did I realize why, soon after the incident, my father bought me a puppy. We brought her to the hospital to meet my mother, who hated dogs. I had never questioned his unexpected gift; now I see that I didn't want to know or remember. With the probable exception of my father, no one else knew what had precipitated this descent into hell. My mother went to her grave not knowing. She could never have grasped or accepted any of it. On his deathbed, the last morning I saw my father, I thanked him for my education and went home to do the laundry. That was barely twelve years ago, yet the impact of that awful night still comes alive in my mind, no less piercing and vivid, but no longer disorienting.

In my adult life before H., in meeting with a string of psychiatrists and psychologists, none of these memories spoke up to say they were tied to my depressions, longings to end my life, low self-esteem, pervasive fear, conviction that I was stupid, inexplicable feelings of shame, need to hide, difficulty sleeping, and a collection of feelings in disarray.

In college I was an indifferent student, except in literature classes, before drifting into a lonely marriage, though one that produced children who brought purpose to my life and gave me, on the whole, reason to live. Still the depressions worsened until one day I called my children's pediatrician to ask for a referral to someone who could help me before I drowned myself. He gave me a name, saying, "I've seen her turn a lot of teenagers around."

This new psychiatrist was a psychoanalyst. I knew little else about her but I recall flying to these visits as if for an oxygen treatment. To pay her without having to leave my children for long periods, I put an ad in the paper and began to babysit in our home while these young mothers played tennis and went out for lunch. I began to feel better even as the marriage faltered. Within a year or so it ended. Lights went on in a movie theatre in my mind, the film had ended, and I was walking out. This time therapy had changed me. I was sure of it. I was starting a new life, depression-free.

Within a year, everything collapsed once again. I didn't understand that depression did not fall out of the sky, but was connected to something within me. This is the point at which this story begins, when I started to see my present therapist, H.

Therapeutic Process

For several years we skirted the edges of my issues; it was support, not therapy. That began to change soon after I remarried. I had begun working indirectly with women who had been abused, and found myself shaken by their stories. It was a time in my life in which the love of my husband and relative job security were offset by the stress of living in a newly blended family that included five teenagers and increasing pressures from my ex-husband. My mind felt like the inside of a pinball machine. Was my therapy wrapping up or just beginning? I felt myself living on two planes: one was the everyday life with my husband, kids, and job while the other was life in the strange space of my therapist's office.

There we slogged through years of my stuff, years of self-loathing and shame, slowly pulling together the stray pieces of my story. I could not understand why he would do such ghastly work. I hated and feared him, yet never missed an appointment. His arrogance enraged me (I couldn't see it was an overlay of my father, a fixed expectation of being hurt), yet I drank his kindness. Our sessions felt like a torture chamber because of the feelings they evoked, therapy a maddening jigsaw puzzle.

Yet he didn't give up on me, nor I on him. He let me set the pace, never rushing me, saying only what he felt would help me. He was the only person who understood me, and I needed that profoundly, as probably we all do. I never had that as a child. All encouragement was withheld in favor of criticism and punishment. Maybe one reason I didn't quit was I loved feeling that someone held out some hope for me; or maybe what happened is that I began to understand myself. His understanding of and compassion toward me became my own.

Growing up in a crazy place is not the cause of everyone's emotional travails, but it turned out to be mine. In the process of therapy, I have made a detailed self-portrait and a fair composite sketch of both my parents. That may not sound like much, but for most of my life I would have been hard-pressed to write a single coherent paragraph about any of us. When I would start to write a sentence about my father, nothing would come out of my pen. When either of my parents entered the therapeutic space I was apt to flinch or twitch, rock, or put up my hand as if to ward off a blow. Bit by bit the ferocity of their visits has lessened.

Sometimes in our sessions I would become distant, and he would ask if I were angry with him. *No, of course not.* It was a long time before I could feel and admit it. My formative world did not allow my anger; only theirs. I had to learn how to do this, with him, and he provided a safe space to do so. Had we delved into my memories without this safety valve—being able to acknowledge anger toward him—I would have bolted. When we began to tap into the memories of what happened, it became harder to hold on between visits, to keep the connection to him, so I began to see him twice a week. Anger and fear, both directed toward him, were odd but reliable ways of reaching the feelings attached to my memories. H. was not the source of my massive anger and subsequent depressions, but he became a lifeline to reach the memories to which they were tied.

Often, as I waited for his office door to open, a faint, odd feeling crept into my awareness. Too insignificant to mention, it persisted from my earliest years of seeing him. I imagined that he would come out of his office and wouldn't know me. This never happened. Year after year he would open the door to usher me in for my session, and he always knew me. Still I had this feeling; still it was never important enough to mention.

Then one day I went for a very early appointment. At this early hour, no one else had ever been there waiting, yet a man was sitting there. I sat down. My feelings began to work on me. Why was this man there? He must have an appointment. He didn't appear to be waiting for the person now in session. It could only be that my therapist had forgotten that this was my time. It also meant that I no longer mattered. There could be no other explanation. I picked up my purse and left, driving the one-and-a-half hours home. Once home, the phone rang. It was my therapist. The other man had shown up at the wrong time. He told him that a woman had been waiting, but she left. My therapist apologized for the confusion, but I was dazed—not, I think now, from disbelief, but from being hurled into a memory.

At our next visit, our talk opened a door to a cache of feeling about the countless times in my life that my mother stopped speaking to me. Ignoring my pleas, she would resume our relationship only when she was ready, without apology or explanation. It was like being annihilated; for her, I no longer existed. This was my mother's way, but my feelings about it were absent—until this moment with my therapist, in a rush of pent-up sorrow. In time, it also explained how even the slightest hint of rejection by someone would pull the rug out from under me. It echoed my early experience. When I explained how often my mother would say, "You always make a mountain out of a molehill," he observed, "For children there are no molehills." To him, my feelings mattered. He never pathologized them or put labels on me, but spoke to me with plain and simple words.

These insights into the workings of my family proved crucial to my emotional well-being. Most were drawn from little incidents with H. This trusting relationship with a personal emotional detective supported me through a maze of feelings to the sunlight of understanding.

Mostly the weather of our sessions was overcast with lots of rain. The hardest parts were facing the fear, rage, and shame of buried memories: the past, which wasn't past at all. The past was as present as kudzu vines choking the life out of a tree.

I learned that many of us who suffer significant trauma in childhood don't develop emotionally beyond those experiences unless someone helps us. We have trouble seeing the therapist as a person separate from traumatic memories of earlier relationships. This was unnerving for a long time, as if there were two planes of reality in my mind, at odds with each other, yet both true. H. was so kind to me, but often I hated him. He withstood the onslaught of my grief and pain. Meanwhile our relationship sustained me in the work, and our visits now are less fraught with ghosts.

Afterthoughts about Therapy

Over a long period in therapy, I read anything I could about abuse, even torture, trying to find my place on the map, the place where my story fit. I wanted something that would help me make sense of myself. Clearly, something had happened in my family, but it was unlike examples I came across in books. In time I learned that it doesn't matter whether we are traumatized in combat, by a parent's early death, an abusive family, rape, betrayal, or even torture. The severity of the experience might vary, but the feelings for us all are the same. No device can measure such experiences, such feelings, nor a void where feelings should be.

A few books have given me a larger perspective. These are books I was drawn to, not that H. recommended. I was well into therapy before such books became relevant to my understanding of the impact of what had happened in my family. About ten years into therapy I found *Trauma and Recovery* by Judith Herman, which I hid from my therapist, as if I would not be allowed to know what it said or that it had something to do with me.

Another book was *Soul Murder, the Effects of Childhood Abuse and Deprivation* by Leonard Shengold. Even knowing otherwise, I used to think of abuse as scalding or cigarette burns on an arm. It is even more than that. Shengold writes, "Soul murder is neither a diagnosis nor a condition. It is a dramatic term for circumstances that eventuate in crime—a deliberate attempt to eradicate or compromise the separate identity of another person…depriving the victim of the ability to feel joy and love as a separate person."[4] That sentence described the family of my childhood. Reading it helped me substantiate what has been extremely difficult to see, understand, and accept emotionally, even as I knew intellectually what took place.

Not a single word of what I have read helped me get out from under the pain, anxiety, and depression. All relief came from the embattled, extraordinary relationship with my therapist. Until him, I never knew what it was like to have someone who believed in me and what that could mean to someone's life. Maybe it's the reason I love working with incarcerated youth. From my own childhood I understand a little about what happened in theirs. One of my students wrote a poem to me entitled, "To This Great Woman"—I'm a volunteer literacy tutor—but it meant that much to have someone who cared about him, however briefly. I am acquainted with that profound gratitude to someone who feels I matter.

Becoming stronger in therapy made it possible to do the difficult work it entailed, and to regroup more readily between sessions. I was learning about myself through a connection to another person. Or, I should say, learning how to have a connection to someone, in this case my therapist, then eventually to other people.

Infants and small children, if loved and protected, glow with an innate sense of trust. In some families it is lost, though we may not realize that our emotional problems are connected to events in our lives that strained or broke our capacity to trust others. Life is much harder for those of us who feel we can't trust anyone. Having a therapist is a way to learn how to feel safe again and to re-learn trust.

Gauging Progress and Benefits

In some therapies people acquire discrete skill sets—maybe reducing bingeing episodes, getting out of habits of negative thinking, or learning to manage anger. The acquisition of these particular skills may be sufficient to get on with living. But to feel alive at all and to think of myself as a person instead of something that should live under a rock, I needed all the skills. For me, it was about how to become someone who wasn't afraid all the time, who didn't think I was stupid, and who didn't feel dead. Therapy was about my whole self. Since it involved all of me, I can hardly begin to describe the ways my life has changed in every part and level of my being.

The back and forth of therapy—not just the back and forth of conversation but also the back and forth of progress-retreat, progress-retreat—can be discouraging and feel like no progress at all. Incorporating a new awareness at first is fragile, tentative. We have to circle back to it many, many times before it becomes ours to keep. I used to call my therapist's answering machine sometimes to hear his voice, sometimes leaving my voice on the tape next to his, just to feel safe again. It's hard to believe I used to need that, but I did.

I have spoken of the great fear I had of my therapist. I knew he would never hurt me as well as a soldier returning from war knows there are no roadside bombs at a 4th of July picnic in Moline, but that is not the message sent from our hearts and amygdala where terror is seared into memory. It rushes in to seize center stage before whatever is real and now ever has a chance to make its presence known.

In the course of our work, his words could conjure my father's presence. Fear invaded me until I could later find the words—my words—to bring emotional control and perspective. Upon leaving his office, I would begin to replay the session. Sometimes on the train home I would write out my feelings, expressing what I couldn't say in person. The pages, bearing the date, disappeared into a box in my closet. Writing out my feelings let me preserve many of the helpful things he said and to sort out my feelings, a little like silverware in the drawer. The urgent need to write was to me another of my symptoms, and an embarrassment, so I kept that hidden too.

But some years into therapy with H., I began to read some of these pages. My father was dying and I felt thrown onto a whirl-a-gig. I was trying to come to terms with this man who was my father. Rather suddenly I was curious to know what I had written about him, and knew where to find it. These pages held clues and insights that I had forgotten in the rush of life. Assembling them chronologically, I saw that many of my issues over the years were no longer issues. This amazed me. I was so accustomed to berating and belittling myself—now I know where that came from—I had hardly noticed that I was making progress, that issues one by one were being settled. I was changing, and I held the evidence in my hands. No longer did it slip and slide. Finding and re-reading years of painful entries, seeing how I had worked through so many of my troubles, renewed my commitment to therapy. I finally saw what it meant to "work through" something: it doesn't bug you anymore like a hornet in a jar.

Alarms would sound in the course of my therapy, and all of them had to be worked out. If my therapist wore a blue shirt like my father, my anxiety spiked. If something in a picture on the wall reminded me of my father, I couldn't concentrate. At other times my therapist might say something that I would interpret as arrogant, again like my father, and I would withdraw from our conversations. I didn't notice, but he did. There is no end to what others might regard as "weird" reactions, but he put these clues to good use, helping me dig deeper to understand why I did things, until I didn't need to do them anymore. "Symptoms" began to fall by the wayside.

All along the way I was ashamed for being a long-term therapy patient—even though almost no one knew I was in therapy. At first it made no sense. Then I began to see that I projected my shame onto others and turned it into what "they" would think of my being in therapy. Whether it is called stigma or shame, the feelings are the same. Now I can see that these deep feelings of shame suffused my idea of myself like black ink. Those ideas about myself were what had to change; they were also what didn't want to budge. The shame was connected to what had happened in my family.

Finding my feelings in therapy was the way out. It was always about coming to understand my feelings, draining off the rage and grief of memories. As we pieced together fragments of the past into an approximation of what happened, I was letting go of symptoms—defenses against knowing what didn't want to be known—I was becoming stronger, more confident, more energetic, and my prevailing moods more cheerful. I see now that all along the way he was quietly, persistently urging me to think for myself, which bit by bit helped me think of myself as "someone" instead of as "nobody."

Ending Therapy (or Not Yet)

I devised a false self to get along in the strange world of my parents. I was asked, perhaps like many children, to make up for their emotional deficits, rendering my absolute obedience to them both. Even in death my father is a beloved and charismatic uncle, brother, and grandfather, but my experience of him was different. The effect of his anger was of a sledge hammer driving a post into the ground. For so long a monolithic fear, and maybe some of it was fear of my own rage, dominated my waking and sleeping life. Inch by inch it is becoming smaller and doesn't wedge its way into my life as it once did.

The relationship with my mother was not held together by tender feelings. She was hard to love. In her quest for perfection she could see only my faults and never shrank from her duty to remark on them. Probably without conscious intent she tried to keep me from ever being independent of her. My guilt at wanting to leave, and surely guilt for hating her, sealed the arrangement. Therapy has made it possible to have a life of my own without having to serve her endless needs even after she died.

My parents were oblivious to the effects of what they said to me or to each other. They saw no harm in words. They couldn't see themselves or see how shut off they were from warm relationships. Neither of them knew an encouraging word, to give or receive. Families like mine keep us from playing all the notes on the piano of our selves, and some notes remain silent a long time. Therapy lets us work out our complicated feelings, the same ones we stumble over, retreat from, and try to avoid altogether.

Trauma and Recovery lists seven diagnostic criteria of complex post-traumatic stress disorder which were under consideration for the fourth edition of the diagnostic manual of the American Psychiatric Association. Whether or not these criteria were adopted is immaterial to me, but I read the list recently and saw a piece of my history in all of them. In the early years of therapy they were only words on the page, not in my heart. It has taken me a very long time to recognize and own them. But my therapist never looked at me beside a list of criteria. I have only been someone with a mess of feelings to be sorted out. Where I saw a big lump of failure, he saw a human being with possibilities.

I have stayed in treatment because I could and because my life runs better with therapy than without it. It's one thing psychologically to be injured by someone outside the family; it's another thing entirely to be injured by a parent, or both parents, and to have their ugly ideas of you embedded in your bones. Without knowing how to be good parents, oblivious to others' feelings and numb to their own, they passed along the effects of their own difficult childhoods.

Simply in quiet conversation, H. takes the little things I say about whatever is going on in my life and combines them to make something nourishing and substantial. We are engaged in an effort to re-shape my ideas about myself. He follows the lines beneath the surface, locating where they are tied and knotted. He knows just where and how to loosen them enough for me to work them free. Without loosening these ties, I would have stayed sealed in the past, as if in a tomb.

When I berate myself for continuing in treatment, I remind myself that these are my parents' voices telling me that I am not worth it, that I have something wrong with me. The life I have now would never have been mine without therapy. I am grateful that I found a therapist who is as constant as the sun and who, by illuminating different aspects of my life, has helped me make sense of my inner world till I could become part of the larger, vibrant one around me.

A friend who was a Navy pilot during the Vietnam War told me that he thinks every day about that time, of those who were lost and those who had to carry on. I believe it is the same with emotional burdens of whatever kind: of those who live with shame, who return changed from war, who want to kill themselves, who have suffered some terrible loss, or who live with the marks of someone's treachery, even their own. I hope this book will encourage them to look to therapy to find a way out of pain and the dark shadows cast across their lives. I wrote it because in the early years of my awful loneliness I might not have felt so different from other people if I had known others saw therapists, sometimes for years and years, or even all their lives, just enough to make it through; to know that someone had found peace and joy because of the relationship with their therapist; or to know there is no shame in it and that it's worth the fear, discouragement, and pain.

So, when depression and anxiety lifted (not naturally like fog, but with steady work in treatment), I began to see that I was not the only person weighted with emotional problems. Others were also saddled with shame. I was clear about the changes therapy had brought to my life: my husband and our family, work and interests I loved, increasing freedom from a preoccupation with something unfathomable in myself. No longer was the idea of suicide my default solution to disappointments and setbacks; no longer did I feel lost in my own life. Somewhere in this period, the idea for this book appeared, as did the man in the waiting room.

The lives that come together in this book are like the characters in a play. Just as in the musical *A Chorus Line*, each person steps forward on a darkened stage to have the spotlight shine on them for a few moments, they tell another part of their story. Then that character steps back into the shadows and another person steps forward. There is no music other than the sound of their voices, quiet and sincere. We read their stories, recognize some of ourselves in each one, and realize that their response to the problems they faced was simply human. Those who find anyone strange or different from themselves are ill acquainted with their own hearts, because these feelings belong to us all. The only real difference is that these few individuals are a cadre of determined people beating back stigma surrounding emotional problems.

Here the conversations about therapy begin.

PART TWO

Conversations about Therapy

Chapter I

Deciding on Therapy

Decide that you want it more than you are afraid of it.

– Bill Cosby

EVERYONE is afraid of therapy, at least at the start. That's why most of us take so long to get around to it. Every person I spoke with vividly recalled his or her decision to go into therapy, no matter how many years had passed. It was that momentous.

Yet notions of why people go into therapy are hazy. In clinical terms—adjustment issues, life stressors, family or marital conflicts, depression, life transitions, etc.—the reasons sound mechanistic. The feelings and stories behind them, outside of psychology textbooks, are much more interesting. How did they decide to go? Did they wake up one morning and just do it? Was something else going on? Would they talk about how it happened?

The interviews started out in a question-and-answer format, but as each of my respondents sat in the quiet space thinking aloud, many ideas reached well beyond the topic of "deciding." A decision implies a precise moment in time. These suggested more of a process, part of something larger and more complex, one that included the gathering of wherewithal—time, money, a therapist, the courage and willingness—to talk with someone about their lives. The process often entailed deciding and re-deciding as the reasons to go and not to go got sorted out.

As each person is introduced, we see just how often "deciding on therapy," "finding a therapist," and "re-deciding" blend. The combinations are so varied that I came to think of the space these "decisions" occupy as a sort of anteroom to therapy itself rather than as a linear progression of discrete segments. It is not uncommon for people to enter and exit therapy several times, especially in the early stages, sometimes with several intervening years, before they finally "decide" and settle in with a therapist. And playing in the background of each person's life are subtle influences tending to motivate or deter them.

Sarah

Sarah saw several therapists before finding someone who felt right, and yet even her unsatisfactory experiences in therapy yielded greater self-awareness. As her confidence increased, her judgment improved. She grew up with her parents and younger brother. Her father was an alcoholic, the impact of which she felt throughout her childhood. Married and divorced by twenty-one, Sarah married again after a five-year courtship when she was thirty-three—but divorced again after a year.

"My first time with therapy was when my brother passed away from suicide. My mom wanted me to go to counseling with her. That lasted awhile, then my mother bailed out. She didn't like what she was hearing and didn't want anything to do with it. But I continued. I was seeing good things from it. Initially it was about how to work through this, but it started bringing everything else out. My father absolutely would not go."

Going in for one thing and coming out with something more is a theme threaded through many respondents' stories.

Sarah went to counseling a second time while dating the man who became her second husband. "We were struggling, and I was still struggling. I had issues that weren't resolved. And to this day I don't know how to go about finding a good counselor, someone who works with you, or where you go to find one. I went with my girlfriend's idea and went to hers. I have really low self-esteem."

She also found her third therapist through a friend. "I liked her. I met Hank when I was still married, and I was hating myself, thinking I make bad decisions, what's wrong with me. A lot of it was self-esteem—thinking badly of myself, thinking I'm not smart. I wanted therapy. I was craving it, so I wasn't in conflict with myself about going. No matter what situation in my life came up, I didn't feel good about the way I handled it or what I thought of myself."

The counseling that grew out of her brother's death changed Sarah's life. "After my first counselor, my progress just kind of sky-rocketed up. I wanted more. I wanted to really change myself. Then I'd have a dip, then I'd sky-rocket back up, then I'd kind of just be in the middle. Now I'm riding that nice comfortable wave where I feel real good."

Through her work with four different therapists, the last two of which included Hank, she felt her life was in a steady state.

Learning about Therapy

Initially Sarah went to therapy after her brother's death. When her marriage failed, she returned. She used it to help her deal with specific situations, and working these out seemed to stabilize her self-esteem. She was not in conflict about going; in fact, she was "craving" therapy. Then she added, "No matter what situation in my life came up, I didn't feel good about the way I handled it or what I thought of myself."

Her comment implies a wish to study patterns in the big picture of a life. Though most of us enter therapy expecting it to be short-term, the truth is that none of us knows what will happen when we go into it. Our ideas tend to be rather vague about what it is and what it can accomplish, certainly about what we need or want, and what we are willing to work for. How could we know? The fields of psychology and psychiatry are complex, and so are we.

To simplify matters—because this is not a psychology textbook—only two kinds of therapy are contrasted here and both appear in rather general terms. The first tends to be solution-based and symptom-focused. As one woman put it, "I feel that therapy is about problem solving of the here and now. I don't want to talk about the past for hours. I want to talk about what's happening to me now, how I'm feeling now, and decisions I'm making, to have a more practical approach to therapy..."

The second kind of therapy tends to be open-ended (though not necessarily longer-term), in-depth, insight-oriented therapy aimed toward personal growth and repair. Many people find a home in this kind of therapy when short-term interventions have been unable to make a lasting difference in their lives.

Even within these loose categories, there are no precise boundaries. Goals often shift. Since no one type of therapy has been scientifically proven to be superior to another, no one type is espoused over another here, though my experience in long-term psychodynamic treatment is evident throughout.

As is my bias; I like to understand people's comments in a context. For example, when she was fourteen the young woman quoted above, who wanted to talk only about what was happening to her *now*, had survived the murder of her parents by a sibling. Raised in a deeply religious family, she went on to say, "The process of recovery is about opening out and helping other people, and not being so selfish." I include her comments as well as a little context not to distort her meaning, but because the context is important. She had spoken of attending a support group in her early twenties. Everyone was "a high achiever and functioning," all in their forties. "But," she said, "they seemed really trapped in their past. For me, seeing them in their forties and still dealing with these same issues over and over again, I said, *I don't want that for myself.* I want to figure this out and make peace with it...so that when I'm in my forties I'll have moved on."

She decided that wouldn't be her fate, an understandable choice. But maybe she never got to see those people five or ten years later, to know that they had been able to—not *put away once and for all,* because we can't—but at least come to terms with what happened in their lives. Maybe those who hung in there are no longer mired in the past the way they were while undergoing therapy's mystifying, cleansing, integrating process. Nor do we have the chance five years later to see the young woman I spoke with.

Given my bias, I have often thought about some of her comments, "You just wonder, if you pulled away the conscious and controlling mind, what would you find there. That's just kind of a low-grade anxiety...I've always tended to intellectualize rather than be emotional about things...One of the residual issues in life is that I don't really allow myself to get angry." Maybe the important point is that she did not want to deal with the old stuff *at that time* because she wasn't ready. Or maybe she didn't have a therapist who understood what needed to be in place before she could even begin to pull back the curtain.

Nearly all of us go in to therapy, at least the first time, to solve a specific problem, then leave. Few go to therapy to understand themselves better by means of insight-oriented treatment, though many end up there. Some of us return to therapy years later to dig more deeply when we feel a need to explore questions of how and why we came to be who we are. The message of this book is that each person has to find a therapist who makes sense to us at a certain time in our lives; my hope is that the diverse experiences of my respondents will prove helpful in figuring out what might be best for you.

Hank

Even before he'd met Sarah, therapy had made enough of a difference in Hank's life that he readily offered to talk with me. He grew up with his parents and sister, married young and had a daughter, Katie. As marital problems sprouted, they went to a therapist for help; Hank went by himself to a second one. Ultimately the couple divorced. Shortly after my meeting with Sarah, she and Hank had begun seeing another therapist as a couple.

Leaning back in a rocking chair in an upstairs room of the house they shared, Hank expanded on why he went into counseling. "I'm very inquisitive. If somebody tells me an answer to something, I have to know how they got that answer. 'How'd you know that?' That's just me. I went because I wanted to find out what was wrong in my marriage and I couldn't find the answer myself."

Then he spoke of his first marriage: "The first time I decided to see a counselor, it seemed my wife and I were continually growing apart. We had a child, and I loved being a family man, but I had to find out why it wasn't working. But with the first counselor it was going nowhere. She'd say, 'Well, try dating, try all these things,' and I'm thinking, 'No, there's a deeper problem than just trying to date and be good to each other.' There was a real problem, and the therapist wasn't getting to it. I didn't know what the problem was, but I knew she wasn't getting it."

Receiving Clear Signals

Intuitive knowledge enjoys high status in our minds, and this clear emotional signal helped Hank decide to see a different therapist. Sometimes emotional currents interfere with signal clarity. Without it, decisions are harder to make. Self-doubt, internal conflict, or disapproval by an authority figure (or entity, such as some religions) are a few of the interferences that make a decision to go into therapy harder for some than others.

Reliable signals, free of interference, can be received based on the degree to which we are free to listen to our hearts and make our own decisions. We shouldn't need anyone's permission to go to therapy, yet disapproval of someone close to us can interfere with our decision, slow our progress, or even kill the impulse to try. So these decisions may be more complicated than we realize.

Christine

On a chilly night in the late fall I drove out to meet Christine at her apartment on the edge of the campus of a large Midwestern university. Seated comfortably at the kitchen table, she began by telling me she had graduated in the spring and was now working at the university while she considered options for graduate school.

She grew up in "a close family" with her parents and younger brother. During her junior year of high school, her mother discovered Christine was bulimic and insisted she go into therapy.

"At first I didn't want to do it at all—you know, the stigma. I was adamant about not going, and she finally talked me into it saying, 'Lots of people go to therapy, and it will be helpful.' I did go and found it very helpful."

Christine's symptoms improved in a few months, but at the end of her junior year in college, the bulimia came back. "I didn't want to tell my mom or anyone because I felt that . . . I felt like a failure. I thought, 'I didn't beat this the first time, it's come back. I'll try to beat it by myself.' I didn't want to admit that I needed help."

The scenario repeated itself. Her mother found out and told her she had to go to counseling again. At first she insisted she could "fix it" herself, but her mother prevailed. Christine returned to the same therapist, someone she had liked very much. "I did better this time because I'm older and more mature. I did that for a couple of months again."

"My mother told me that it's normal for people to go to therapy. She said it would help me with the bulimia and with other problems, too. I was feeling sort of depressed and was painfully shy. I worried about what everyone thought, like the imaginary audience. I thought everybody was looking at me all the time and judging me, and my mother had said, 'The therapist will help you with your self-esteem, the bulimia, the depression. It will help you in all these facets, and you'll be happier.' So that's what clinched it for me, because—not in just one area—therapy would help me in many.

"I went to the therapist, and she asked me if I was on any antidepressants or if I had been to a psychiatrist before. She said that it might be a good idea to go to one and just see how it is. So I went to the psychiatrist at the campus health center. She was very nice and helpful and gave me Prozac. That has helped me out a lot, too. I never really thought about taking antidepressants before, and I'm glad I did. Even my mom noticed after a couple of weeks that I was happier.

"I felt disappointed about seeking help because I've always been an overachiever. I set standards for myself that I don't set for other people. The conflict was that I couldn't do it by myself. I was disappointed with myself, like a failure.

"I didn't tell my friends that I was going to a counselor. I would make up little excuses, like a doctor's appointment. Eventually I told one friend, then another, and I felt better after telling them. It was sort of like a weight off your chest, and I didn't feel stigmatized at all. They were very supportive and friendly and open-minded. And some of them, I found out, had gone to counseling, too! And I was, like, 'Oh! I'm not the only one!'" she laughed. "I guess the stigma prevented me from sharing it at first, but not anymore. I'm much more open and easygoing about it.

"What precipitated going was pretty much my mother finding out about the bulimia. If she hadn't found out, I don't know if I would have gone." I asked her how her mother had discovered that the bulimia had returned. The first time she had purged in a bottle in her room, and her mother had found it and confronted her. The second time, her mother found similar evidence. Both times Christine tried denying the truth—in fact, lying—and both times her mother kept probing. "So she knew, and she wasn't going to take any crap from me," she added tearfully.

She went on to describe some of the feelings that made her wonder whether she wasn't "as happy as another person would be." In high school she was valedictorian, Fourth of July queen, and prom queen. "All these wonderful things happened to me, but I always felt less of myself. I was unhappy, and I don't think I knew it at the time."

Overcoming Reasons Not to Go

Christine admits the unlikelihood that she would have gone to a therapist without her mother's insistence. The appealing prospect of being helped not just with the bulimia but with depression, shyness, and the negative feelings she harbored about herself, overcame her initial resistance.

Her remark, "I was unhappy, and I don't think I knew it," echoes in other stories. The comment reminds us that we all go in to therapy thinking we know ourselves more or less—how could we not?—only to discover that actually we don't.

NIMH Eating Disorders and Other Illnesses

Eating disorders...frequently coexist with other illnesses such as depression, substance abuse, or anxiety disorders...People with anorexia nervosa are 18 times more likely to die early compared with people of similar age in the general population.[5]

Greg

Greg had also seen a university counselor when he was in his last term of graduate school, though our conversation took place many years later. We met for a few hours one rainy Sunday afternoon. He talked about his experiences with therapy, which he had used just enough to get himself up and running again.

When he was a teen, Greg's parents divorced. His father moved across the country and remarried, while Greg continued to live with his mother and younger sister. In graduate school he had been under a lot of pressure that suddenly dropped off. "I had just a few classes that were real easy, and I couldn't even do that little bit. I thought that was strange. I was handling all the hard stuff—then had a little let up on it and had a hard time getting my homework in. So I went to a counselor at the university. It was just a few sessions, but it was useful."

He said that another time he and his wife were in couples counseling to deal with issues in their marriage. "There had been just enough therapy in my life that it was a normal thing to do when you need help."

Some years later, his mother was diagnosed with Alzheimer's, which gradually engulfed her in depression and confusion. "We needed therapy for her when this all started. We knew someone who had a good therapist, and he recommended a psychiatrist who works with elderly patients. I started taking my mother to see him. I would just sit outside, so I wasn't in on the sessions, but she would go in on her own and talk.

"In the meantime I was under more stress, taking care of her and seeing her go downhill. It was hard to see her lose all her independence. I was getting depressed and could feel it weighing on me. So I went to this same doctor because I thought, 'Well, he already knows the situation, knows my mother and what's going on.' I started to see him once a week.

"It had mostly to do with my mother's situation, and I don't know that the doctor . . . he didn't do tests or give me a diagnosis, but it was obviously a depression. I guess I probably could feel it. Things weren't fun, just kind of feeling down all the time, not being able to get as much done as I had hoped. My wife noticed it, too. You could see—anybody that would know the situation would see—the problems with my mother.

"It was a little bit of a hassle. Most doctors you go to once or maybe go back a second time. This is something you have to do—in my case, once a week—so it's something of a hassle to schedule and keep up with it." This was on top of a demanding job.

Recognizing Depression

It interested me to hear Greg say that "it was obviously a depression" and in the next breath seem a little dubious with "I guess I could feel it." It is an example of one of the many guises depression wears—apparent to us at times and other times not. For this reason, self-administered questionnaires available on the Internet or at the pharmacy to determine depression are not the whole story. We may be emotionally numb, unaccustomed to thinking psychologically, or imagine ourselves immune. Or, sometimes depression sneaks into lives on cat's feet.

Many people are unaware that depression may underlie conditions for which they seek medical attention. Some family practitioners and pediatricians are alert to it and know how to screen for it, but, there again, many people refuse the diagnosis and turn to another doctor who tells them what they would prefer to hear. Still others accept medication for the depression but do not seek therapy. Or, some people say that being depressed is a "choice" people make. No one would *choose* to be depressed, but perhaps it is a choice by default if we do nothing about it.

NIMH People at Risk of Major Depression

People who were abused or neglected as children have increased risk of major depression, which often begins in childhood and has lingering effects as they mature... Previously abused or neglected study participants with depression were also more likely than matched control participants to meet the diagnostic criteria for at least one other mental disorder, such as post-traumatic stress disorder (PTSD), drug dependence, dysthymia (a less severe form of depression), or antisocial personality disorder.[6]

Allen

One day a man who had seen a copy of my "Dear Someone" letter called to set a time to meet, saying he felt strongly about the importance of reducing stigma. When Allen arrived for his interview, we laughed at how secretive we were about our therapy. His wife had nudged him to call me, saying, "She's going to have trouble finding people." Because nearly everyone I interviewed had seen more than one therapist, participants began with an overview of their history in therapy. Allen's route was more direct than most people's.

He grew up with his parents and two younger siblings. After his first marriage ended in divorce, he married his present wife, Sharon. He saw his first therapist for a year, and then was in family counseling with Sharon for a few ye ars as they sorted out matters of a remarriage when both spouses have adult children.

He happened to read an article in the newspaper about agoraphobia, written by a psychologist. It rang a bell, so he saved it. Feelings of social anxiety had plagued him, and he had "tried to cope in my own way for thirty years."

He recalled his first experience with panic, when he was in college. "Up until that time, in social situations—going places, traveling, doing whatever—I hadn't encountered any unusual difficulty . . . but I can remember distinctly sitting in a study area at college with three or four of my buddies talking—about baseball, whatever—and I became fearful, just a panicky feeling that I can't ascribe to anything . . . an almost overwhelming feeling of terror. Panic. Feeling trapped in that situation, feeling a terrible uneasiness." The feelings subsided, and "life went on."

"But then, as time went on, panic attacks occurred again and again." Sometimes they were associated with a situation in which Allen might expect to feel somewhat anxious, like public speaking. At other times, when there seemed to be no threat at all, panic could overwhelm him. Sometimes he had to excuse himself to find a men's room to vomit.

As years went by, he would have to travel on business to give presentations. One night in his hotel room, even knowing he had done his best to prepare, he couldn't sleep and broke out in a sweat. "I don't know whether the chemicals involved finally ran their course, but all of a sudden there was a release." The sweating stopped, and he could sleep, knowing everything would be all right the next day. And it was. But the feelings of impending disaster were so overwhelming that he felt he should find a therapist. Still he put it off.

Not long after, he was asked to go overseas, where he would face a language barrier and work with people he hardly knew. "That whole assignment terrified me so bad I couldn't do it. I had to tell my boss, 'I'm not going to be able to cope with this.' And then I had to explain why, that I had these feelings of anxiety, and so that was the first time I had to share with him."

"I felt in conflict about seeking help. 'Why can't I cope with this, see it through, bite the bullet, or even, being a God-fearing person, why is it that my faith alone can't get me through this? Am I just not enough of a believer, that with my faith and help from God, that I can't overcome this?' In my training, you measure this and you measure this, and things many times dovetail. There's an explanation. The practical part of me said, 'You ought to be able to put all of this together and cope with it and do whatever you need to on your own.' The social expectation was that a man ought to be able to handle these kinds of things and figure it out. 'You ought to be tough enough to punch through this on your own!' I'm sure those factors were what took so long for me to get off the dime.

"There's no question that the stigma of having mental health issues was part of it. It was much easier to understand a physical limitation. If you tear a ligament doing something and then you can't play a certain sport, it's a physical limitation that has no stigma. It's just something that happens. But mental situations . . . . 'You ought to be able to control that from within!' That's what mental is about—it's your brain power, it's your perception of things. To me there was a stigma attached to not being able to deal with things that other people—other men—have no trouble with.

"The stigma of a mental problem versus a physical problem was in my mind a very big difference. 'I can't control the physical changes that take place in me, but something involving the brain—I'm in control of my thoughts and feelings, aren't I?'

"Not totally, evidently, I've come to find out!" he laughed. "'I'm feeling this way—isn't that something I have control over?' I found out it's much more than that."

Before his problem worsened, Allen called the psychologist and author whose article he had saved. He told his boss that he had found a therapist in the area who dealt with phobias such as this, and his boss understood. "He was a wonderful boss. Very understanding." Allen was lucky.

My guess is that when he speaks of the stigma of not being able to do "what other men do with no trouble," he speaks for legions of men. We think we are the only ones who are afflicted by some condition that, to us, is inexplicable. Nearly everyone I spoke with voiced this concern in one way or another.

Acknowledging Stigma

Except in certain circles—among therapists and fine novelists—the complexity of our emotional life is kept largely under wraps. We keep our emotions that way so we can press on with daily life. Also, many of us grew up in families that didn't allow for difficult feelings such as fear, anger, and jealousy. They didn't know what to do with them. My theory is that the difficult feelings, which make up "complexity"—the feelings that some of us have trouble acknowledging in ourselves or expressing—contribute to the stigma associated with mental health concerns. Unable to talk about the difficult feelings, the problem becomes what to do with them. Eventually they are crowded out, or so we may think.

The stigma associated with unpleasant feelings warrants a closer look. Any stigma that goes unchallenged is strengthened. When we look away instead of standing up to it, we allow the stigma that accompanies psychological ills to gain the upper hand. We hardly think about what it means, individually and collectively, to bow to stigma's control over our lives.

Here's one. A subtle stigma thrives in the power of pharmaceutical companies that influence our idea that pills can solve just about anything, from attention deficit hyperactivity disorder (ADHD) to erectile dysfunction to obesity. The primary goal of the pharmaceutical industry is to sell a product and make profits. Hardly anyone tells us that therapy can also be helpful—even *more* helpful, and certainly more durable—but we are primed through relentless advertising to think of pills as a solution.

Stigma makes a subtle appearance in a newspaper obituary for an eighteen-year old who "died suddenly at home" of an "accident." It is as if we all know and tacitly accept this stigma. The focus of articles or conversations shifts, leaving questions unanswered. This may be out of respect for the family's privacy, or to divert a copycat effect, but perhaps it also perpetuates a little white lie we accept to keep ourselves from the profound mystery and pain of suicide.

When an employer, with kind intentions, suggests an employee might consider therapy to help with problems that spill over to work, it's stigma in action when the employee responds, "I'm not crazy!"—implying that therapy is only for those who have gone over the edge. When a number of doctors over a period of several years suggest to a patient that depression underlies her condition and she flatly dismisses the idea, perhaps that is stigma too.

Both Christine and Allen have mentioned stigma. An awareness of it appears in many of the comments among these stories, yet it barely crosses the minds of others. Why? For some of us, it is as if the stigma itself is unbearable. Why? Maybe stigma is worth thinking about, for its faint trail winds among the reasons to avoid therapy.

NIMH Anxiety Disorders and Depression

Anxiety disorders, such as post-traumatic stress disorder (PTSD), obsessive-compulsive disorder, panic disorder, social phobia, and generalized anxiety disorder, often accompany depression.[7]

Nora

Some while after I met Allen, a friend put me in touch with Nora. She had gone into therapy to improve the relationship with her school-age daughter. Nora's original family included an older sister; her father, who was starting his own business when she was young and thus was often not at home; and her mother, "who was a complainer."

She recalled feeling as a child "that I really didn't have anybody there for me." She mentioned having read about mothers like hers, who have postpartum depression and who don't want to touch their children. She thought, 'Is that my problem? That lack of closeness?' "I'm always wanting to cling to somebody, I tend to get too close, then expect things back, and make it the close relationship that I didn't have."

Nora married at twenty-three. After her daughter's birth, her mother came to help, but Nora "wasn't that thrilled" about the impending visit because she feared she would be taking care of her mother, which proved to be the case. During that visit she confirmed that her mother was an alcoholic.

Some years later, Nora became close to an aunt who lived nearby and who was in therapy. When Nora expressed her distress at not getting along with her daughter, her aunt recommended the therapist she was seeing. Nora's daughter, Maureen, was also willing to see the therapist, and they saw him separately each week for a year.

"My daughter and I were not getting along. I couldn't understand why she was acting the way she was. The therapist would say, 'Quit running in to solve the problem. Let her solve her own problems unless it's life-threatening.' I would always try to make her happy and couldn't understand why she wasn't. As much as I tried, I was concerned for her and for our relationship. Something wasn't right."

Nora recalled her feelings about therapy. "I've always been curious about what makes people do things—it's fascinating. When my mother went through shock therapy for postpartum depression with my sister and me, she saw a psychiatrist. When I was taking a class at school and said, 'Oh, wouldn't it be cool to go to a psychologist?' she said, 'No, you don't ever want to do that.' She felt that it was not a positive thing if you needed help."

Nora did not adopt her mother's view. "I looked at therapy as an opportunity to get some help with my daughter. I was curious to find out what someone else would think about what I'm thinking."

Embracing the Promise of Therapy

Nora has taken a direct path into therapy: problem, referral, appointment. How easy is that? I wondered if she had experienced previous trials where some therapy would have been helpful, but one question I neglected to ask of my interviewees was this, "Do you recall times when you might have wanted to consider therapy but turned away from it?"

Consider the influences around us that give therapy short shrift. Advertising and marketing by pharmaceutical and insurance industries, some churches, and government programs, along with comments of friends, try to persuade us that medication, motivational reminders, seven visits to a therapists, or diligent prayer should suffice. It's as if it's just a matter of keeping a positive attitude, just a matter of deciding, and then simply shaking off those pesky feelings! The list of ways to achieve inner peace is nearly endless: survival in the wilderness, meditation, massage, yoga, fasting, and countless others. All of them work for some people, but not with equal durability and strength.

People avoid therapy not because they don't need it or wouldn't benefit from it. Many learn to live unremittingly on the surface of feeling. Or they keep themselves busy every waking moment to keep their feelings under wraps. Many pass along to their children a reluctance to deal with such issues, as if we don't want to talk about *that.* Or things aren't *that* bad. Or we put the blame on someone else. We avoid therapy not because we aren't miserable, but because we can't bring ourselves to face what needs to be faced.

A key role of a therapist is to support us while we face what we try hardest to avoid. Any therapist knows it takes uncommon courage to face unwelcome truths about ourselves and sometimes about others we are close to. It takes courage to return to painful memories we thought were buried once and for all. It also takes uncommon persistence when our memories won't yield their feelings on demand. Sometimes it's hard to stay the course when our very own therapist seems to be so annoying. Perhaps they are, and we may need to seek out a different therapist. Often, though, we need to ask, "What is that about? Is there something here that I'm avoiding?"

Many people wait too long to look more closely at themselves to ask, "What is going on here?" This is played out in headlines every day. They tell of suicide, murder, domestic violence, road rage, depression and numerous other psychological ills. Such headlines hint at stories of people overwhelmed by their problems. We may wonder about their decision not to ask for help in time, but for each of them, that would be another story.

James

James was a casual friend I'd known for several years. I had told him about the project I was working on and one day asked if he knew any men who would let me interview them about their therapy. To my surprise he offered to talk about his own experience. Soon afterward we set a time to meet.

His partner, Daniel, had undergone a long hospitalization from a serious car accident, and after that, James began to accompany him to therapy. They needed help with the changes that resulted from Daniel's brain injury. James struggled not only with guilt about the accident, though he had had no part in it, but also with questions about what he wanted in his life and what he had the courage to face.

"I was having trouble separating myself from the situation I found myself in, which was having the courage to still be a part of Daniel's life without being his partner and lover, and opening up the possibility that I could have something for me independent of that—a new relationship, or just being on my own, or doing something. That took a lot of courage. That's really what started me in therapy, and it took a long time for me to realize that the best thing for him and for me was to move on."

He stayed with Daniel for four years after the accident. "To this day, I am still a part of his life, but it's better for him that I'm not in that situation because I was resentful. I felt like I was half of an old couple dealing with very serious illness that you would find later in life, that you just resign yourself to.

"I wasn't in conflict about going to therapy because I was going with my partner. When I decided to see the therapist on my own, I didn't see it as a weakness. I respected my therapist, and one of the first things he said to me was that people who are more 'together' or more in tune with their lives tend to be people who want to seek help. And the people who are unwilling or unable to see things in their lives that they want to change are clueless. They're not strong people." If James was uneasy about being in therapy, his therapist made it okay.

Seeing Things We'd Like to Change

Few of us who want to go into therapy have someone who encourages and points out that it's an act of strength. There are many more whose problems with alcohol, broken relationships, anger, depression, excesses, intractable debt—the list is long—but who may not see things they'd like to change in themselves. We are all more objective about others than about ourselves. And, as these stories illustrate, until our problems become "bad enough," we find plenty of reasons for not considering therapy. The shoe really has to pinch before we take it off.

More readily they might consider therapy because of a specific problem, then find that "the problem" is attached as if with silken threads to other parts of themselves such as their values, sorrows, and longings, and these too deserve attention. When no part of us is excluded, the whole self is enlarged in addition to solving the initial problem.

We begin to see that no matter what the issues are that any of us bring to therapy, it is an opportunity to reflect on our lives in a way that gives clarity and meaning to our experience. We see ourselves in a different light, and that self-knowledge is freeing.

Melanie

Melanie was referred to me. When I called and we chatted awhile, she said she was well acquainted with the stigma of psychological matters. We set a date to meet. In a light and airy apartment overlooking a train station, the afternoon sun fell along a row of plants lining the window ledge. She had prepared steaming cups of tea to sip while we talked, and became quiet only when the occasional train roared by.

She described her family as one in which her father "was in charge of everything" and her mother "just did whatever he said." Her mother entered a long period of depression when Melanie was in the fifth grade "where she hardly ever got out of bed," and family members vied for attention.

Her family frowned upon therapy, so "it was a hard decision to go." Before deciding on therapy, she sought support through religious faith. At that time she was in a physically abusive relationship with a boyfriend and felt she was having a breakdown. Someone in a group she had joined recommended a therapist whom she saw "for quite awhile," but stopped because "it wasn't working for me anymore, and she was not being helpful."

Melanie hesitated for a few moments, then continued, and more details emerged. It was a reminder that my quietness made room for *her*, which was the point.

She had seen the first therapist for several years before stopping. "My sister was also afraid to go into therapy, so she saw the same person. That ended up causing problems, and now I know why. I'm sure it was very exciting for the therapist to be able to see the whole family dynamic, getting two different perspectives, but it ended up re-creating the same situation that I had in my family."

Melanie continued, "I was so insecure when I first went into therapy that I couldn't even get a decent job. Having therapy enabled me to feel like I am worth getting paid to do some work in my life. It had a profound effect on my life the first time around. I did get a certain amount of pride and self-esteem that I didn't have before, and I moved into a competitive field and did pretty well. Before therapy I didn't have any ability to do that."

After a dozen years without therapy she resumed with a different therapist. Self-esteem issues lingered, and they interfered, she felt, with her ability to have lasting relationships. Things were "still just not working out." She had "a couple of very unusual negative run-ins with some girlfriends," and she "lost a couple of friends and was having a hard time dealing with that." A friend who was in therapy suggested that she might want to try again, and her friend's therapist had the wisdom to recommend a different therapist.

Going into therapy was easier the second time. She has been seeing her current therapist in the hope of improving her relationships with both men and women. Although self-esteem and relationship issues brought her to therapy both times, her focus the first time was on establishing herself in her field. Some years later it shifted to deeper issues: "When you're looking for the ability to hold down a job, you're talking about a level of self-esteem that's easier to attain. But when you're looking for something where you're starting to deal with big things about your personality, it's more difficult."

Stalling Around

Melanie's first experience with therapy, which she thought had been going well, was derailed because of the therapist's poor judgment in allowing another family member to become a client. Eventually Melanie came to terms with the experience, came away feeling stronger and better able to make her way in the world. But her first therapist's professional lapse contributed to Melanie's postponement of therapy and, in essence, may have cost her several years of a life less burdened.

Most of us are thrown into therapy by a crisis—just when we are least able to do the necessary work to find a truly good therapist. And most of us don't know how to find a good one or what "good" means. We usually call the first name that comes our way, at the most desperate point, when all our other efforts to solve our problems have failed.

I have often wondered why we stall around. We seem to exhaust every other possibility, keep our head in the sand, avoid acknowledging how difficult things have become, reject any suggestion that we might be even a tiny bit depressed or only slightly anxious, pin our hopes on a "physical" diagnosis or on medication—anything to avoid seeing a therapist (or taking our child for help).

Despite the popular idea that the "stigma of mental illness" exists in the society around us, the longer I stared into its face the more I came to believe that the actual stigma is more within us than it is outside us. We are ashamed of needing help and we vehemently do not want to face the causes of our disease. Instead we don't get around to finding a therapist or find someone or something else to blame for our unhappiness.

Claire

Through word of mouth, as happened several times, I received a call one evening from a woman named Claire. Shortly after that she drove out to our house, I brewed fresh coffee, and we settled down to talk about experiences in her life, including therapy. She came to the United States from England and had made her life here without any family.

Before our meeting she had written a poignant reflection to serve as an introduction to her comments:

> As a child I believed that the world I inhabited was how things were supposed to be. Whatever happened, I did not question it. I assumed that because I was treated badly I must have deserved it, and I believed that if only I could just be better behaved, do better at school, etc., I would earn my parents' love and everything would be right. As an adult I struggled with depression, believing this was inherited from my mother. I developed crippling migraines and muscle spasms in my body so painful that it often made it hard just to get through the day. I put those problems down to genetics as well. I was puzzled at my inability to have a successful relationship with a man, but kept trying anyway. Finally, at the age of 40, after one more disastrous relationship, I gave up the struggle. I resigned myself to spinsterhood, a life of celibacy, and determined to try to find happiness in some yet to be determined way. Only in my late 40s and 50s did I discover that children and adults do not have to live this way, and that was what I felt my therapy did for me.

Growing up, Claire didn't think anything was the matter with her family. She believes now that she was always trying to conform to its norms. At one point the family moved, and her mother started going out to work. "For whatever reason, my parents started having fights. They'd scream and shout at one another. My mother would throw things—not my father—and I remember being scared a lot of my childhood. I took care of my brother because my mother worked long hours. My father was a teacher and came home about the same time as we did. I spent most of my time with my father, and he and I were responsible for the housework and laundry and cooking. In retrospect, I didn't have much of a childhood.

"I think I learned to survive on my instinct. My mother suffered from borderline personality disorder, which is where somebody either completely withdraws and is unavailable to you or is so up in your face that you want to slap them. It was very unstable because I never knew what to expect, whether it was going to be one of the close times or one of the times when I was to keep away. Even at a very early age I learned to live very much on my intellect."

Claire enjoyed being at school, away from the tensions at home. She excelled academically and liked visiting the homes of her friends. At eighteen she went away to college and had her first serious episode of depression. Her internist's recipe for recovery was to "wait until the spring and you'll feel better when the sun comes out." Instead, she left college, went to live in London, and lived "a pretty wild life for a few years." During this time she became pregnant. After the delivery, she relinquished her baby for adoption.

"You didn't really have an option about keeping the child, because it was a stigma for both mother and child. I went into a deep depression after I had the child, but, as I said, you didn't have depression in those days. Nobody went on pills or for therapy—that in itself would have been a stigma."

In her twenties, Claire moved to the United States: "At some level I knew I needed to put some distance between me and my dysfunctional family." But a few years later she experienced another serious depression. She believes she didn't seriously try to kill herself, that it was "just a cry for attention," but she took an overdose, and then called a friend, who took her to the hospital. A psychiatrist saw her there and referred her to a psychologist for therapy. Over time she was helped to see some of the reasons behind choices she had made.

She stopped therapy and went on for a few years that included "a lot of disastrous relationships with men." Her job took up so many hours of each day that she couldn't think much about her personal life. Even when a friend observed that she wasn't much in touch with her feelings, she thought, 'What does she know?'

One day, after a series of bad relationships, she felt as if she were going into "a dark well that went on forever, with no way of stopping and nothing to grab onto." She sat at her desk at work, thinking about people she knew who were in therapy, who talked about it, and she thought, 'I need help, because I don't think I'm ever going to climb out of this place unless I do it.'

"I was picking the wrong men, or they were picking me, and I felt that something was wrong with me. There were episodes of mental blackouts where I'd be on the bus riding home, and I'd end up twenty stops from where I was supposed to get off. I was blacking out and knew at some level that I was in trouble. I felt that if I didn't seek help I was going to be in even worse trouble. I had to get to the root of my problem.

"Up until I crashed and burned, as it were, my life was pretty good. I was active socially. There were a lot of things that I was interested in and doing. But there was always an underlying feeling that something was the matter with me, that I'm not the same as other people."

Noting a Few Lessons from Therapy

Claire was only one of many people I spoke with who recalled not being able to remember details they felt should have remained in their minds. At the time, they were unable to see how bad they felt or the ways in which they ignored feelings that had been there all along. Emotional problems can be like their physical counterpart. The longer we wait to do something about them, the longer our bodies and minds accommodate themselves to disability and limitations in unhealthy ways that stifle creativity and sap energy.

Nearly everyone remarked how much better they felt about themselves and their lives because of therapy. This was in contrast to their apprehension at the outset. Yet I don't want to convey the idea that therapy is a cure-all, as if people achieved a pinnacle and stayed there. Rather, they learned about themselves, put feelings into words, and came to understand some things about themselves they had dismissed or overlooked. Often they needed to work to maintain an ongoing awareness of tendencies to slip back into old habits.

Throughout these stories we can see how easy it is to think we—any of us—are being honest with ourselves, only to discover how carefully we avoid knowing what we don't want to know. With the intriguing mind/body connection, we learn more about the ways our bodies express psychic pain. We see examples of ways the unconscious mind directs our conscious life, as if by an orchestra director below the stage whom we can barely see or hear. Meanwhile, some denounce the maestro, whereas others cultivate a relationship.

By pondering an idea of ourselves, as shaped by genes and family dynamics, we see how that idea can be modified and redeveloped in close relation with a therapist. We see that in the process a person's age is largely irrelevant, that in our inner world time exists outside of calendars and clocks—a memory just as vivid today as six or sixty years ago, awaiting our return and willingness to settle matters. We also consider why it is important for a therapist to have done his or her own work in therapy. Altogether we see how it is possible through therapy to find a way out of psychological conditions that, like a tourniquet, constrict the flow of feelings and keep us from enjoying life more fully.

Rose

Rose and I met in her home one summer afternoon. She was seated on a yellow sofa in her living room, leaning against some bright pillows as she began to talk. I sat nearby with my tape recorder resting on a small footstool. As with every person's interview, I have read Rose's comments many times, and each time some new facet catches my eye.

Rose's father died rather suddenly when she was a young child. A year or so later her mother married a man Rose already knew and liked. Her father's good friend had come to their house to play cards, and she remembers that "he used to take nickels and quarters out of my ears and do all these sweet things." But she also remembers that her mother's relationship with them both was "stormy."

A crisis in Rose's marriage was the impetus for going into therapy. But she saw the therapist only four times, then stopped because her husband didn't want to continue. She returned the following year, seeing this therapist for several years until she went back to school, substituting college for therapy. Some years later she returned for another few years, stopped, then resumed, and has since continued without interruption.

"Going into therapy was not an agonizing decision—it was the next logical step. I was in a bad situation. That's when I picked up the phone. That was the beginning of when I started to go, and it was probably once a week, then it got to be a couple of times a week. I had no money. They saw people on a sliding scale, so it was very inexpensive. But I knew people who were in psychoanalysis, so I just thought it was the next step. I don't remember feeling like it was a bad thing to do. I was proud of it. I was taking care of myself."

After years of stop-and-start with therapy, Rose became very sick. Illness prompted her return to treatment. "I was feeling very defeated . . . I felt I had some responsibility for an illness that I didn't understand. There were enough people saying that it was due to unresolved grief, so I went back to my original therapist. Most of my therapy and analysis has been with one person, and it's been for most of my adult life."

Bearing Responsibility

Rose was the only person who described her decision to go into therapy as "the next logical step." It seemed to be related to her awareness of other "people who were in psychoanalysis," so perhaps going herself was an extension of what was already a "logical" and normal thing to do. This is an example of the relative good fortune of being in a community that places high value on sound mental health, and for whom seeing a therapist is as natural as breathing. For too many others, it is an "agonizing decision," one with an aura of stigma.

In another comment she said, "I felt I had some responsibility for an illness [this was a physical condition] that I didn't understand." It seemed possible in the logic of her soul that her illness was due in part to unresolved grief over her father's death. No one else but Rose could make her take care of herself; she had to see the need, wonder about it, and do something.

Jenny

Some months after beginning work on this book I was talking with a lawyer I met at a conference. In our conversation he happened to mention having done "a close study of the effects of trauma." This chance remark stayed with me. It seemed possible that he might be able to put me in touch with someone who would be willing to talk with me. So, many months after meeting him, I called him and explained what I was doing. He seemed interested. Shortly after that, the phone in the kitchen rang, and it was Jenny, who had a story to tell. We agreed to meet the Saturday before Mother's Day.

The day brought warm temperatures and sun, and when Jenny pulled into the driveway, I went out to meet her. She was soft-spoken, blonde, and gracious. Sitting at the kitchen table for awhile—we both admitted that we were a little nervous—she shared some of her story with me.

Her father, an alcoholic, left when she was three years old, and her parents divorced when she was six. Her mother quickly remarried; a year later her father married a woman Jenny had known all her life. She and her older sister lived with their mother and new stepfather until she was twelve, when they divorced.

During those years she was the victim of repeated abuses by members of her family. In her twenties she married and was divorced, then married her present husband, with whom she has a son, age six at the time of our meeting. After that brief introduction, we went into the living room, turned on the tape recorder, and spent the afternoon talking.

"My mother, without fail, put herself and her needs before mine or my sister's. She had psychotic episodes, but with the narcissism, she would be doing her hair, getting ready to go out for a date, and if it didn't go right she would throw her hairbrush at us and call us 'fucking bitches,' screaming at us because her hair wasn't going right.

"My stepmother tells me that we were always sent to them dirty, looking like little waifs. I've done a lot of reading, and my mother fits the definition of the destructive, narcissistic personality. All narcissists believe that the world revolves on its axis around them; destructive narcissists want to destroy you if you do anything that counters that belief. I've always been afraid of her wrath. And for a long time it controlled me."

Jenny made "a few weak attempts" at suicide when she was twelve. "They were really cries for help. My mother screamed at me and threatened to throw me in the loony bin, and then ultimately took me to a child psychologist," but she recalls being unable to engage with him.

Fifteen years later a crisis drove her into therapy once again. "I had broken up with a boyfriend, and he came back, waited for me outside my apartment and raped me. That was a watershed moment for me because, thanks to God, something in my mind clicked and said—I'd had several bad relationships prior to that—'You know, you're choosing these people. You can either live your life alone or find a way to change yourself so you're not choosing people like this.' And that's what drew me back to therapy." However, she found the therapist was not helpful, and I did not press her for details.

At twenty-six, she married—"I married my mom"—then fell into a serious depression and was referred to a clinical psychologist, "the first person I ever trusted at all." After a few years he told Jenny that his wife was seriously ill, and he would have to stop practicing to be with his kids. She later learned that he didn't quit his practice but merely dropped her as a patient, breaking her fragile trust. Soon after, Jenny's marriage ended.

Around this time she had begun seeing in tandem another psychologist because of his expertise in Eye Movement Desensitization and Reprocessing (EMDR).[8] Over the course of a few years she missed as many appointments as she kept, because the memories threatened to overwhelm her. To find a way to keep going, she would commit to just six appointments at a time, and then commit to six more.

Jenny remarried and gave birth to an infant daughter who died within a few days after her birth. A few years later a son was born and she saw the psychologist a few more times. "But I didn't keep it up. It was too hard." When her son turned two, Jenny returned to therapy with the same psychologist. "I was afraid of turning into my mother, and I was feeling a sense of responsibility with regard to my stepfather being out there somewhere continuing to hurt children." She set out to find him and to "let the people around him know what kind of monster" he was.

At the time of our conversation she had seen her therapist for perhaps ten years, including interruptions. She laughs, "I get sick of him every now and then, and I take a break—I say, 'I'm sick of you, I'm sick of me, I'm sick of my stuff!' and I'll take a month off, but I'm still actively seeking therapy." Since working with her therapist she has had to recommit to therapy several times "because it's been such difficult subject matter and such intense emotions." Then she added, "There's something inside of me that compels me forward to try to heal from this."

After several hours we stopped with the intention of resuming in a few weeks, but all the interview excerpts were taken from that one meeting. She had brought with her many pages taped together till it was three feet long. On it she had recorded in chronological sequence a series of violent events at the hands of her sister, mother, and stepfather. These included being repeatedly beaten and raped by her stepfather, having him urinate on her, being beaten, strangled, and smothered by her sister, and being abused numerous times by her mother. Though Jenny and I have met a few times for breakfast since then, the interview questions were never completed.

Reaching a Turning Point

We don't know why Jenny didn't engage with the psychologist when she was twelve, though it is common that those who are abused hide from the knowledge of what happened. The abuse, though it may be suspected, goes unidentified or unreported. Those who were abused don't begin to address what happened until—or if—they are in the hands of someone they may eventually grow to trust. The slow process of remembering is extremely painful; if the feelings are short-changed, life must be lived with a part of ourselves cordoned off from the rest of us.

Most of us combine elements of wishful thinking, good intentions, and old-fashioned determination to avoid taking notice that difficult feelings have gotten the better of us. We keep ourselves very busy (and distracted), sign up for a self-improvement program, enlist a treatment that virtually guarantees results in just six weeks (or your money back), or seize on the cause of our symptoms as definitely physical—and sometimes these efforts bring the desired relief, at least for awhile.

But when the results turn out to be less than durable, our expectations can wither with the next crisis. Individuals often don't seem to reach a turning point until then. Jenny called it "a watershed moment." Until that time, many of us aren't ready to deal with the issues. Once we reach that turning point, when we are able to think of our situation from a different perspective, we are urged on by a combination of feelings, stresses, crises, and opportunities that cause us to take action.

Beth

Beth, a practicing therapist, was completing her doctoral degree in psychology when we met at her office to talk. Several plants, soft lighting, and comfortable furnishings lent an air of quiet security. A box of Kleenex rested on the coffee table between us.

She described herself as a late bloomer. However, once she decided to go into clinical social work she began working faster than planned on her credentials to become a therapist. At the time of our interviews she was completing graduate work in addition to working in her private practice. In the light of a late winter afternoon we sat and talked as she described her decision to go into therapy for the first time.

"It gets tricky about why I sought therapy, because the first therapist was one of my professors when I was getting my master's degree. I went to her to talk about career goals. I was working at my first social work job at a residential facility, and it was extremely difficult.

"I went to talk about how to manage the job stress, get better at what I was doing, what direction I wanted to go in my life. Never had a conscious thought, 'I'm coming to you for therapy.' And I wasn't! I did not set up an appointment for therapy. It was to help me like a mentor, maybe offer some supervision, which is very common in our field. We might have talked about different directions I wanted to go in my program, and I believe I was kind of, 'Yeah, but . . .' to a lot of things she was saying. I think she brought up therapy.

"She gave me a couple of different names, and I remember sheepishly asking her, 'Well, what if I work with you . . . ?' Not embarrassed, but maybe shy. I believe that's how we set up our appointment, and it was so out of my conscious awareness that that's what I was doing. Maybe I could not bring myself to say specifically, 'I'd like to come and see you for therapy.' I don't know why I wasn't able to do that."

Beth went on to say, "That's how, unbeknownst to me, I ended up seeking therapy. There were things going on in my life—not at a crisis point, but I was feeling incompetent at my job, overwhelmed by it, struggling, and uncertain. That kind of uncertainty makes me very vulnerable. Around the same time I had moved into a condo that had thin walls. I had intrusion all around me, and I developed horrible sleeping problems that went on a few years. It took on a life of its own about feeling intruded on and how do I assert myself. It pushed me into more of a depression, starting with the sleeping problems, lying in bed with racing thoughts. Seeking help was due less to a crisis than to a beginning awareness of something that was in the back of my mind."

Here I was struck by Beth's reference to "a beginning awareness of something that was in the back of my mind." She will show us where it led.

"Consciously I was not in conflict about it at all, but unconsciously I was very much in conflict, so I developed this plan—in hindsight I see that—of how to get what I want without really admitting it or saying it. It was fascinating because it was so unknown to me. Once I was in therapy, it wasn't a problem. It was hard to make that first step, so I didn't. But I found a way."

Taking a Step

Beth describes her "decision" to go into therapy. She sidled up to it as if through a back door, only later realizing how uncomfortable she was with the idea—even as she was studying to become a therapist. (Apparently none of us is immune.) She needed to approach therapy for herself in the guise of wanting to be mentored through career choices, for that was more acceptable.

We observe her awareness of the unconscious realm of her mind as she recalls: "It was so out of my conscious awareness that that's what I was doing. . . . Because I had no awareness, it must have been something that was making me uncomfortable, and I didn't want to realize that...That's how, unbeknownst to me, I ended up seeking therapy."

She was completely unaware that she was uncomfortable with the idea of therapy for herself. For her, reaching a turning point about therapy was due less to a crisis than to a "beginning awareness" of something in the back of her mind.

Summing Up

For each of my interview participants, the decision to go into therapy was part of something larger and more complex. Often the decision came at the end of a series of failed attempts to work things out themselves or upon acknowledging that the problem wasn't going away.

In these accounts were plenty of reasons aside from money not to go to therapy. Sometimes it was not that a person wasn't "strong enough" to do it; rather it was impossible to imagine how much one's life could be improved by talking with a therapist. Others were in conflict about going. For some, seeing a therapist just felt more "normal" and acceptable than it did for others, or "stigma" stood in the way. Sometimes the prospect of what had to be faced was too overwhelming (though a sensitive therapist helps make it manageable). Others didn't realize how unhappy they were, that they were depressed or their lives had become constricted. Sometimes someone close to the person disapproved of therapy or even forbade it. Sometimes people didn't realize that a trial-and-error process of deciding and re-deciding is a typical pattern.

Others needed time to gather the wherewithal—emotional and material—to seek treatment.

There were also plenty of reasons for deciding to go. Sometimes curiosity was a driving force, wanting to know why things were the way they were—or were not—working out despite great effort. Often a crisis precipitated action, though sometimes the impetus was an unrelenting awareness of something being amiss. For a few, the clarity of hindsight helped them see recurring patterns of depression, failed relationships, sleeplessness, or other problems. A few others were encouraged to seek help, and that made a difference. Sometimes a decision was made easier when an opportunity, such as a trusted referral, presented itself. A few others went initially out of concern for someone else, then realized they had matters of their own to discuss.

These interview excerpts about deciding (and re-deciding) to go into therapy illustrated the need to take responsibility for one's own life. They also described ways in which talking about all sorts of feelings with a caring listener can help us understand ourselves and find the means to make some changes.

All twelve of the respondents described how they decided on therapy—some in crisis, others in frustration—but all in need. In the next chapter they talk about finding a therapist. As individual as their stories are, when blended together they also begin to have a lot in common.

Chapter II

Challenges in Finding a Therapist

I saw the angel in the marble and carved until I set him free.
- Michelangelo

WE all want a therapist who will set us free—of guilt, anxiety, depression—all of it. Finding that therapist is stressful and challenging. Early in the search uncertainty clouds the picture. How tempting it is to call the first name you find and be done with it. Or to fall back on a ranking of therapists on an Internet database. Easier yet, simply give up. Choosing a therapist, while easy and straightforward for a lucky few, is a delicate matter. On this leg of the journey, be prepared to park your bike for a while as you sit on a bench to think about what you need and want. If this is a new endeavor, this step is even more critical.

A woman told me about her teenage son who "had issues" following the death of his father. A well-meaning school-counselor recommended a psychologist in private practice. The referral appeared reliable and the boy saw him for a year, missing as many appointments as he kept. Neither mother nor school—nor boy—saw improvement. The therapist confided to the mother that he had told the boy "nearly everything I know." This approach wasn't useful. A close family friend suggested a different therapist, and despite a long weekly commute by public transportation, the young man never missed an appointment. As he began to come to terms with his loss he no longer needed to act out his pain, and within a few months had begun to regain a steady course.

The search for a therapist may be hampered or eased by a variety of favorable and unfavorable influences. The process is dynamic and complex, like everything else about us. We bring as individuals a great deal to the search process without being aware of it. These include tendencies from our families (or religious training) to think positively, get over it, or move on, various folk adages about how to conduct our lives, or an idea that therapy is only for people who "need" it, possibly linking being in treatment with being "mentally ill." Attitudes may have been shaped by a previous experience of therapy, by our degree of willingness to learn something about ourselves from another person's perspective, or a host of other influences. Some will read at length about psychological and adjustment issues to bolster their conviction that they don't "need" therapy while others might step into a performance of happiness and well-being for the therapist's benefit. Others bring with them a belief that human beings can be reduced to four dimensions such as introvert/extrovert, optimist/pessimist, etc. All of these tendencies subtly affect our decisions to go to therapy, to question and wonder, to stay or leave, to judge ourselves (or a therapist) too harshly and prematurely.

Personal qualities like persistence and self-esteem can override discouragement in finding a good fit with a therapist, but what we bring within us to the search process can enhance or sour the experience. This suggests reasons to do some spade work in preparation to receive what will grow in your garden so you don't get rutabagas instead of raspberries.

Obvious Challenges

Obvious challenges—unlike the ones that lurk within us—can be confronted and often remedied. For most of us, the first of these is how to pay for therapy. Like food and fast cars, money tends to be freighted with other meanings. At a practical level is not having enough; at a psychological level is what money may represent such as status, security, power, and control. Either way, "money" can hold us back from finding a therapist.

Many of us find a way despite limited means. We trim our budgets, work extra hours, use community resources, or start with a support group. Even with the benefit of health insurance to cover a portion of therapy, some choose not to use it. Many of those who have found a way to afford therapy have had our earning power increased and satisfaction with work enhanced. Therapy became a priority at whatever cost.

Because so many people who say they can't afford therapy do find a way, the question arises whether sometimes the money issue is a smokescreen for being unwilling to undertake the rigors of therapy. It often entails learning what we don't want to know or remembering what we want to forget. To bypass the discomfort, sometimes people are adamant about being unable to afford it, or we stay with a therapist who doesn't make us work.

Before we have begun to experience a single one of therapy's benefits, however, it is hard to believe that something so intangible might be worth the necessary sacrifices.

Another challenge is the quantity of information on the subject. You don't have to read very much of it to realize the misconceptions you have about different kinds of therapists or the efficacy of certain therapies over others. You might check a few websites, say, about depression, not realizing that the subject you are dipping your toes into is wide and deep. A lot of information floating around about therapy and emotional disorders is superficial at best; a lot is hard to understand. Finding reliable sources is a significant challenge to overcoming doubts and steering your course. A good source is by Kate Scharff, MSW, author of *Therapy Demystified: An Insider's Guide to Getting the Right Help (Without Going Broke).*

One false idea floating in the mainstream is that friends are as good as therapy. Though similar, they are not the same. We cannot place unlimited demands on our friends. A friend might become incensed at our "irrational" anger, but a therapist will stand by us and help us sort through the debris. An exasperated friend might call us "needy," but a therapist will look beyond superficial traits to help us address issues that will strengthen us. Someone who believes that friendship and therapy are the same has not experienced a productive therapeutic relationship. With friends we have an expectation of mutuality, but good therapists do not lean on their clients and patients for help with their problems.

Another challenge is the vast array of confusing therapies and terms; these make it hard to sift through assorted and extravagant marketing claims. Literature that smacks of slick advertising and marketing lingo is a warning flag.

One obstacle to be wary of is opposition from someone close to us; it can be a powerful deterrent to seeking help. One woman's attitudes about therapy, based on a single unfortunate experience, caused her to discourage her unhappy daughter from seeking help; the father of another young woman was so opposed to therapy, he forbade her to talk about him with the therapist she was seeing for depression; and yet another woman explained that she was quite sure she was fully aware of her own mind, that there was nothing about herself she didn't already know. Any of these attitudes can be revised in the course of treatment, but they can also contribute to a disappointing experience.

Subtle Challenges

The search process also may hold subtle or hidden challenges. Among hidden obstacles are depression's flattening symptoms, a sense of shame or stigma, sensitivity to the castigating language and labels that appear everywhere, the effects of trauma which cause us to be unwilling to revisit the pain, staunchly embracing an idea that you can fix yourself, or sticking firmly to a belief that time heals all wounds, to name a few. These obstacles are harder to see in ourselves, though many reappear in the interviewees' stories. Because of the layers of complexity in any of us, even being well informed, well connected, and having financial wherewithal afford no guarantee of success.

In *Psychoanalytic Psychotherapy* Nancy McWilliams says that if change were easy and people could work out their own problems, they wouldn't need psychotherapy. She writes, "It is not uncommon for an individual coming to treatment to have exhausted friends, relatives, teachers, doctors, and spiritual counselors in an effort to solve some intractable psychological problem. And often, these failed sources of help have behaved with impeccable intelligence and concern, only to confront ultimate exasperation in the face of someone's incomprehensible resistance to change."[9] We need someone who can help us overcome our resistance.

Conditions that Make It More Difficult

These include a lack of knowledge and experience in how to begin; how to figure out what you need and want. It's harder if you have no one who is supportive or whose good experience with therapy serves as encouraging testimony. It's harder if you are unable to see you have a problem, if you tend to minimize its impact on your life, or if in your heart you are simply unwilling to do something about the matter. It's also harder if you aren't linked to a community or an individual who understands the value of mental health and therapy.

My intention is not to wither anyone's hopes. If there seems to be an emphasis here on hurdles to finding a therapist, it is because my awareness was heightened as I talked with people and reflected on my own experience. There are many sources of negative messages from the world around us, and just as many reasons within us.

Conditions that Make It Easier

You might receive a trusted referral or know someone who is connected to quality mental health providers. You might have a friend or neighbor who is supportive. Having enough money and a willingness to spend it on your emotional well-being are also helpful. Being within reach of a well regarded therapeutic community such as a college health and counseling center is a boon, as is being willing to interview more than one therapist to find someone who feels right. Being miserable and desperate helps, too.

This odd mixture of complicating factors is why it takes courage to go for help. All these messages swirling together can extinguish a small flame of hope. We may not realize how any of these factors might get in the way of finding a therapist and—even if we find a good one—staying until the job is done.

The men and women in this book chose different kinds of therapy. The therapies varied in duration and usefulness, as did vague expectations of how long it would take or what could be achieved. We seem to gravitate to one kind of therapy or another. An individual's conflicting needs and wishes mix together with the conflicting theories—and, yes, fashions!—of schools of psychotherapy to further confuse the choice.

Finding the right therapist can fall anywhere in a range between a fortuitous referral and an anguished learning process. We usually land somewhere between, and along the way we are strengthened and our judgment is honed, each experience informing us about who we are.

For all the reasons listed here, this is not a "how-to" chapter. How could it be? Rather, it's a preview of what you may encounter. Interviewees tell how they chose their therapists, sometimes why they chose one (or one kind) over another, and some of the obstacles they overcame. "Finding a therapist" overlaps with deciding to go, locating, interviewing, evaluating, trying, and then committing to someone. Paradoxically, we will see-saw between trusting and evaluating the therapist until the relationship becomes better established and relatively secure.

An awareness of others' experiences in therapy may help you shape your ideas and expectations. Even if you end up using a succession of therapists, you are learning about yourself. However, two or five years of seeing a succession of therapists is not equivalent to being in a close relationship with a very good one for that same period of time.

Sarah

Sarah worked with four or five therapists over a period of several years. Yet in our conversation she had burst out, "And, as usual, to this day I don't know how to go about finding a good counselor, someone who works with you, or where you go to find one!" She echoed most people's frustration, almost as if somewhere it was known how to do this, but the elusive knowledge had escaped them. In the beginning none of us knew how, yet by persevering we all found our way.

Sarah found her first counselor through a suicide support group in her hometown. She found a few others through friends, and one through a psychiatrist she had consulted for medication.

I asked her how she and her mother initially found the group following her brother's death. How did they know where to turn? Unable to recall, she called her father and was surprised to learn he was the one who had searched out the group—yet he had refused to go. "He said he needed someone to talk to and he thinks he found the number in the phone book or newspaper. He left the director a hundred messages and finally someone else called him back. People who have suffered with losing someone or have depression really have some deep hurt. I felt it in his voice, just briefly discussing it."

I could imagine that fragile moment of reaching out for help—perhaps he simply lost faith because of the long delay in getting a call back. For whatever reasons, Sarah's father never got professional help. Nearly ten years after her brother's death, the conversation with her father stirred painful memories for them both.

I wondered whether her experience in therapy and her habit of self-reflection had eased her passage toward a measure of acceptance of her brother's death. I wondered if the memories were more difficult now, still, for her father than for her. I hoped to understand if her father had become closed off from that part of himself that held the feelings about the loss of his son, and if Sarah credited therapy as the reason she and her father were in different places of mourning her brother's death.

The decision is enormous to reach out for help following the suicide of someone you love. Sarah and her mother went to counseling and so began the first steps on the long road toward learning to live with their loss.

Being Unwilling to Revisit the Pain

If you are looking to change something in yourself or to work through something difficult, even a short-term situation, therapy can be painful. That's the price of relief. If we could figure it out for ourselves, we wouldn't ask someone else. Pain is a reason to avoid therapy; even if we're in it, we avoid talking about what is painful. For this reason people will find ways of not finding a therapist, not committing to anyone, putting it off, and not getting around to it because of more important items on their to-do list.

Sarah's mother withdrew from the process, which might have discouraged Sarah, but instead she found the conversations in therapy helpful, "seeing good things come from it." This last point, when placed on the scale, helped her decide in favor of continuing despite the pain.

Hank

When Hank thought about obstacles in deciding to seek help for his troubled marriage, he recalled, "I was determined to figure it out. I needed to know. I knew I couldn't do it on my own. Part of the reason I didn't feel any stigma about it was because my mother had gone for help when I was growing up. It was just for help. It wasn't because she was a bad person or because she had a bad problem—it was nothing to be embarrassed about." Hank's mother didn't realize at the time that she had given her son a gift by making it *okay* to go to therapy.

Hank was frustrated by his first counseling experience, and one of his friends recommended a second therapist. "She was very harsh in a lot of ways, but she was realistic. What she taught me was that my ex-wife had a very low-level anger for me and I didn't know why or what I had done, but it boiled down to there being no communication between my wife and me about feelings. She shut down if there were any issues and I couldn't get anything out of her. I didn't know what I was doing wrong. It got to a point where we were so far apart . . . It was like a light bulb went on when she said there was this low-level anger. That was exactly what it was. Then I started realizing why. I began to see what I was doing wrong, but my wife would never tell me. She would just act mad—but I didn't know why. It hit me pretty hard, but I got it right away. We saw this person individually and as a couple once a month. Sometimes every other week—it varied with our schedules."

Hank and his first wife subsequently divorced.

Validating a Decision

Hank was determined to figure out what had happened in his marriage. Two experiences helped validate his decision to see a therapist. One was a memory of his mother's therapy and its positive effect on the family. The other experience was something a therapist said that caused a "light bulb" to go on in his mind. This helped him achieve a crucial understanding about an aspect of his crumbling marriage. Even though the first therapist they saw wasn't helpful, he found another, and although she was "harsh," her insight was valuable.

Sometimes people give up when their decision to go into therapy isn't validated soon enough. It can be hard to figure out whether the person or "therapy" or "the therapist" is somehow insufficient, and many people perhaps give up too soon on one or the other. It's also true that some people are unable to consider what part they contribute to an unsatisfactory experience. But it seems fair to expect to have one's choice of a therapist validated fairly early on in the relationship. If no therapist ever seems to meet one's standards, that is a point worth thinking about.

Christine

Christine had several things going for her when she began therapy. Her mother was clear that her daughter needed help, so she wore down Christine's resistance and persuaded her to go. Her mother also knew of a good therapist in private practice. When the eating disorder recurred a few years later during college, Christine had ready access to a quality student counseling center where her former therapist was in practice, and that worked in her favor as well.

"Finding a therapist was very easy. My mother works at the university so she knew my therapist, who specializes in eating disorders. My mom said, 'I want you to see her because she knows what to do.' That made it easier.

"She's very open and friendly, and I never felt like she was judging me—she always smiled and it's so easy to talk to her. I was so afraid when I came the first time. I didn't know what she'd be like, but she was just a nice woman. The second time I went to her in college, she wasn't disappointed or anything. When I would say something, she would always ask another question, and it would make me think more. She helped me understand why I was doing things; she'd always ask just the right questions. I would be uncomfortable in group therapy, sharing with lots of people—I would be hesitant to volunteer any information.

Christine couldn't have known at the outset that she would gain traction so quickly, but she dug in and put what she learned to good use.

Easing the Way in Finding a Therapist

For the lucky ones, finding a good therapist is easy. In Christine's case we can see the various ingredients bubbling together in a stew of feelings: not wanting to see a therapist, a keen awareness of stigma, a belief she could fix herself, and depression dragging down her self-esteem. But added to the mix was her mother's insistence and continuing support, a conviction that a therapist could help her daughter with depression, self-esteem, and shyness as well as with the bulimia, plus having access to a very good therapist. Several influencing factors made it easier for Christine to go into therapy—yet just as easily she might have avoided it. Although her decision was relatively free of external obstacles, she had a fair share of internal ones.

Allen

It is possible to put off getting help for a very long time. We think, "It's not that bad" or "I can work this out myself." Allen waited some thirty years, though he is hardly alone in his reluctance. Still, once he resolved to get help, he made quick work of it.

"I read an article in the paper about this doctor's interest in phobias, so that's how I came to see him for therapy, then saw a second therapist for a different matter. I was led to him through insurance with my employer. The process was to call this central place and get approval, and they listed several psychiatrists and therapists in the area. One group of therapists happened also to be in the same building where my wife and I had done some family counseling, so I chose someone from that group."

Minimizing Our Problems

On one side of the scale Allen had the benefit of insurance, the name of a psychologist who took an interest in phobias, encouragement from his wife, and a good previous experience with therapy. Yet he still had trouble getting around to therapy for help with his panic attacks. A voice on the other side of the scale seemed to say, "It's not that bad." We also know from comments in the previous chapter that stigma weighed heavily on him.

Perhaps stigma would be lessened if there were support in our culture for those who don't hide the fact of being in therapy. Certainly being in therapy acknowledges that since we are working on some of our issues, we must have a few. Maybe people want to believe that if you are *not* in therapy, you don't "need" it. This idea is simply not true. It is closer to the truth to say that most people, whether in therapy or not, become highly skilled at concealing their emotional problems, especially from themselves. Those who are willing to disclose that they have sought therapy open a door for others.

We lack sufficient objectivity to see the ways our lives are modified because of emotional problems. We discount the probability that these modifications to our lives wouldn't be necessary if we'd find out what is behind them. Once he decided to go, Allen readily found a therapist. But he put it off for a very long time.

NIMH Relationship of Substance Abuse and Mental Disorders

Other research projects show that substance use disorders are often a consequence of primary mental disorders such as anxiety or bipolar mood disorders, which often begin in adolescence or young adulthood. Intervening with the primary disorder may help prevent the subsequent development of drug abuse. Although mental disorders and substance use disorders often appear together, services for them are often separate. Study findings highlight the importance of integrating services for people with comorbid mental and substance abuse disorders, particularly among those with serious mental illness who may be less able to seek appropriate help.[10]

Nora

"How do you know what it is you need? How do you know that the person would suit you? If you go to the doctor for strep throat, you get a pill, and you don't have to go back. With a therapist, you need to go back for a length of time, on a regular basis, and have to set aside time to do that. If I had to go now, I would try to get a name from my family physician; hopefully they have resources."

Being Open to Learning

People's capacity and willingness to confront situations in their lives differ widely. Some of us grow up in a family that tends to "move on" and ignore the elephant in the room; others learn how to face discomfort by growing up in a family that makes it safe for each member to speak their truth, thus encouraging emotional honesty. Probably no one can confront all situations with equal gusto. As far as the relationship with her daughter was concerned, Nora was able to confront the issues between them. She had curiosity on her side, a willingness to ask a family physician for a referral, and an attitude of openness to what she might learn that would help a situation that had been tense for awhile.

Melanie

Therapy was frowned upon in Melanie's family, making it hard at first for her to go. A crisis motivated her to resume treatment after exiting several years earlier. Finding a new therapist wasn't easy, but she did so with less fear than the first time. "A girlfriend who was seeing a therapist suggested that maybe I would want to try again. So I called her therapist, who recommended another person. She said, 'Even if you're friends, and especially if you're another family member, you shouldn't see the same therapist.' It's common that your friend is going to recommend their therapist, and it's so difficult to pick a therapist. You can't pick them out of the newspaper."

Overriding Someone's Disapproval

Melanie's story lets us see the entwined influences that helped her decide to return to therapy with someone new. On one side she had her family's disapproval echoing in her mind, plus a previous negative experience with a therapist who had accepted her sister as a client. On the other side of the scale Melanie recognized how helpful her first experience had been, admitted there was more she wanted to do in treatment, and trusted the friend whose solid referral helped her override any lingering reluctance.

Worth noting is the origin of our ideas about therapy. Both Melanie's family and Nora's mother had given therapy a negative cast. This suggests that even in this area our families instill deep-seated ideas about therapy. It might explain why some of us are open to it and others are not; those early lessons with trusted teachers are all but indelible.

Claire

Claire spoke of her decision to seek therapy, "I had a friend who had been in therapy and shared some of the benefits of it, so I was already halfway there in knowing that it could probably help me. I don't think I would have done it if someone hadn't encouraged me; I don't know if others don't do it because they don't have someone who encourages them. Maybe some people weren't as lucky as me to know other people that had had therapy and that it could help them—or I've experienced people who don't know they have a problem!" she laughs.

Claire, too, had someone who made it okay for her to go into therapy. Next came the matter of finding a therapist.

"I had worked at a volunteer organization with a woman who was a clinical psychologist, and I called her. She recommended a couple of people who I interviewed, and I ended up with the therapist that I went to on and off for several years.

"I only knew that the therapist who referred me thought highly of him—and I thought highly of her. My impression of her was that she was both ethical and caring. If she recommended him, he must be okay. It didn't really matter to me what kind of therapist he was. I didn't know what it was going to take to get me well, and I was not comfortable in the whole therapy situation when I started.

"As I got to know him I learned he was someone who had come from a troubled family himself and had sought therapy, and that was how he had got into the field. He was a very kind, caring person, and in a way he was almost a parent to me. He did the parenting that my parents never did in terms of helping me set boundaries, which was a lot of my problem. He was somebody who was very sure of himself, had very clear boundaries, and could be both stern and kind."

Benefitting from Someone's Support

With Claire we see how dynamic the process is between opposing forces in her head voicing their opinions. On one side is a supportive friend, a connection through a volunteer organization for a possible referral, and a willingness to conduct a few interviews before deciding. But on the other side she admits that even with a problem that was not going away, she was not comfortable at all with therapy when she started. She could have bailed at any point; she could have decided to "tough it out."

A popular idea is that to be successful in life we must be tough, must move on through difficulties, must soldier on no matter what—as if to stop long enough to feel would have us awash forever in self-pity. If we are not allowed to feel, or don't allow ourselves to feel, we risk becoming numb to feeling, living by our intellect alone, out of touch with the messages from our hearts, and alien to our inner life. Sometimes denying our feelings by "thinking positively" or "moving on" makes it harder to work through those feelings later. Our true feelings don't just go away; they are part of us. The challenge lies in understanding them and keeping them more or less manageable. The role of a therapist is to support us as we try to become more skillful at it.

NIMH Depression's Relationship to Other Medical Illnesses

Depression also may occur with other serious medical illnesses such as heart disease, stroke, cancer, HIV/AIDS, diabetes, and Parkinson's disease. People who have depression along with another medical illness tend to have more severe symptoms of both depression and the medical illness, more difficulty adapting to their medical condition, and more medical costs than those who do not have co-existing depression. Treating the depression can also help improve the outcome of treating the co-occurring illness.[11]

Rose

When Rose was strapped for money, she used community resources to get therapy. Her cousin knew about the tensions in Rose's marriage. "My husband and I had had this huge fight, and I started telling her that I wasn't sure he was going to come back, and I didn't know what we were going to do. She was in therapy and told me to call. It was several social workers in a group practice.

"My husband and I went four times. He said he wasn't going to keep going, and I said, 'If he's not going to go, I'm not going to go.' I was twenty-six. A year later, some good friends of ours were in marital trouble. My girlfriend was calling me every day and crying. But my own marriage was in a state. That's when I picked up the phone."

Rose told the therapist what was going on in her life, and added that she couldn't understand why her friend called her when her own life was such a mess. "I remember what he said when I called him: 'Just because you're having problems yourself doesn't mean you can't help somebody else.' That was the beginning. It was probably once a week, then a couple of times a week. I had no money. They did see people on a sliding scale, so it was very inexpensive."

When Rose describes the first meeting with her therapist, she feels an immediate connection. He seems to understand something about her, perhaps illuminating a wish in her to know herself more deeply.

"My therapist is like no one I knew. Physically he's kind of powerful looking without being intimidating. I do remember the first time he walked out to greet me that I felt very small next to him. The first time, I was sitting and waiting for him and he came, and I may have been a little intimidated, but when I was giving him my history and told him about my father, I said, 'Well, my father died—but I was only five years old.' He looked at me and said, 'Only five?' What did I know? It was my mother's loss, it wasn't my loss. I was only five."

So I remember that first session giving me something to think about. I brought him this picture of my current life, and in fifty minutes he was helpful."

Feeling a Connection

Years later Rose still remembered what the therapist said to her. The memory of his words and kindness helped her call for an appointment. She briefly saw one other therapist, but most of her work in treatment has been with one person.

Helpful once again is the image of a scale that weighs the influences of whether or not to go into therapy, whether or not the right therapist has been found. On one side, she had "no money" and, in spite of a marital crisis, her husband refused to go to counseling. On the other side, a reliable referral came from a cousin she trusted. From previous interview excerpts we learned that she knew people who were in psychoanalysis and felt "It was a good thing!" to be taking care of herself. But perhaps most decisive was the immediate connection she felt to the therapist.

Even though she put off therapy for a few years, the impact of that first impression persuaded her to return.

Jenny

Jenny has a lot of experience in the school of get-over-it. Her father would say, "All you need is hard work," as if hard work would make her feel better.

Because of him, part of her still believes depression is something that people give in to because they're weak. And she has internalized the message that people shouldn't need therapy or medication to be un-weak—"Just be un-weak!"

Thinking of Jenny, I could imagine how much my courage would be undermined to have such an idea instilled in me at an early age, especially from a beloved parent, how long and hard I would try to be un-weak. Alongside the feeling that she must be weak is the problem of not knowing where to begin to look for a therapist.

"You're not going to look in the phone book for something this personal. If they're dealing with issues of shame, which so many of us are, it's not like they're going to ask their neighbor, and maybe won't even bring it up with their family doctor. Even if you do, or you get a recommendation from a family member or a friend, it might not be the right fit. Also, people need to feel free to reject a therapist, if it's not a good fit. You need to know that there is someone out there that *will* work!"

Believing Therapy Can Help

Among other influences, Jenny was swimming against the current of her father's attitude. To make things even harder, a sense of shame kept her from bringing up the issue with her family doctor. Yet determination rings in her voice—feeling free to reject a therapist who isn't a good fit coupled with a belief that "There is someone out there that *will* work!"

Permeating our culture is the sense that therapy should be something we do out of necessity, only if all else fails, as if we should hold out as long as humanly possible. Also, should we succumb to therapy, it's a sign of strength and valor to get through it as quickly as possible. Given Jenny's history of abuse, it hardly seems possible that anyone would tell her to buck up, or that she could expect it of herself.

Looking at therapy another way, it could be said that as long as we still feel ourselves changing and growing, deepening our understanding of events in our lives, becoming better able to cope with challenges before us—to be more fully ourselves, to feel our lives being enriched, and to feel ourselves being more open to life—therapy has value and meaning. Therapy is neither a race nor a business; it's a relationship we form with someone who, we believe, can help us heal and grow.

NIMH Mental Disorders and Adult Role Disability

An NIMH-funded study finds that more than half of U.S. adults have a mental or physical condition that prevents them from working or conducting their usual duties (e.g., role disability) for several days each year, and a large portion of those days can be attributed to mental disorders... Nationwide, [over a one-year period], about 2.4 billion disability days resulted from physical conditions, and about 1.3 billion disability days resulted from mental conditions... Estimating the impact of specific diseases on disability is difficult because people tend to have more than one illness or disorder at a time, such as depression and heart disease. [12]

Beth

While she was a student in clinical social work, Beth sought mentoring with a professor, an experience that turned into therapy for a few years and then stopped. Some years later she resumed treatment, this time with another therapist. Most of the following comments concern her second therapy. The interview began by my asking how she chose to study psychodynamic therapy as opposed to other kinds and to choose the therapist she did.

"Because I'm going to school and learning certain things, and those are the things that make a good therapy, with my second therapist I wanted someone who espoused those same philosophical ideas. I wanted someone that could work with the forces within a person, like the unconscious, and the ways we do things that on the surface might look and seem one way but there's a host of other reasons and motives beyond a person's behavior. That behavior is multi-determined, and what you see is not always what you get. I didn't want an approach that would just look at the surface.

"I wanted to understand a lot more about myself, in addition to just fixing it. I felt that the longer term cure was in the understanding, not in the fixing. I wanted someone who had that same philosophy—who wouldn't give me homework assignments, who wouldn't want me to write down pros and cons. You know, tape some affirmations on the mirror. That's all helpful, but obviously there's something about that that's not working for me, whatever that is. So I wanted that deeper approach.

"What I like about [my second therapist] are two things. She asks me what I make of things—to understand things in more depth, and what comes to mind when I'm talking about some of these things. The other piece she does is if I'm talking about something, and she'll have some association to something based on what we've talked about, she'll share that with me. It's not in an intrusive way, but I feel like she's having a reaction to what I'm saying, and her reaction will help me understand more.

"My first therapist was very different from my mother, for whom everything would be a big deal—'Gasp!' With this therapist, nothing was a big deal. Things were able to be talked about, and nothing shocked or fazed her. By that I'm not meaning to suggest at all that she wasn't emotionally engaged or present. But it was such a difference from my early experiences where everything was a big deal. She could hang in there, and we could talk about whatever.

"And my second therapist is like that, too, but because I had that experience—I was so aware of it, hungry for it, and attentive to it—now it seems like it's kind of worked itself out. It's important, but I say to myself, 'Well, she *should* be able to hang in there with me!' Now it's the expectation that people are able to hang in there—it's legitimate and valid."

Wanting to Know Yourself

Beth contrasted her two experiences of therapy. In the first, she was figuring out what she wanted and what was reasonable to expect; in the second therapy she was well on her way toward a doctorate in psychology. As a therapist with an established private practice she also had a deeper understanding of what she wanted in a therapist—someone who would look beneath the surface at forces in the unconscious to understand how they determined her choices and behavior. She wanted to understand herself.

Beth understands that we have a deep reservoir within us that is largely unknown to our conscious awareness. She also knows that not everyone can, needs, or wants to dig around in there. While not all therapists are trained to work with clients at that level, and some specialize in one treatment approach over another, many therapists blend their approaches to suit a client's needs and personal goals.

Summing Up

Being aware of the influences that aid and hinder the search for a therapist contributes to a better informed choice. The interview excerpts illustrated ways in which these various elements are weighed in participants' decisions. Obvious challenges were money, a confusing array of therapies, and someone's disapproval; subtler ones were the ways depression tends to undermine our efforts to get up from the mat, a sensitivity to the stigma of being in treatment, and a deep-seated unwillingness to revisit painful memories and feelings, perhaps choosing instead a numbing agent, such as alcohol or food, relentless busyness, or buying sprees.

Some conditions made it harder to find a therapist. These were a lack of knowledge and experience in knowing what you might want (or need), having no one in your corner who is supportive, being unable to see you have a problem, or living someplace without links to a community or individual who is sympathetic to a life troubled by emotional pain.

Yet some conditions made the inevitable challenges easier. Among them were receiving a trustworthy referral, having someone in your circle who is supportive, having enough money to afford therapy and being willing to spend it on your emotional well-being. Being miserable and desperate, patient and determined also helped.

These influences, favorable and unfavorable, were woven among the stories in this chapter. We saw when a decision was validated by the memory of therapy's positive effects on the family of one's childhood, or something a therapist said that felt exactly right. Being convinced that one's problems are "not that bad" can stand in the way for many years before admitting that a problem is not going away; meanwhile the fulfilling aspects of one's life are greatly diminished. Some people seized the opportunity to "get some help" with a difficult situation; some accepted help, but only to a degree and then they exited. Many had to override the disapproval of someone close to them; more fortunate others had someone's unwavering support.

When the search process entailed interviews with a number of therapists or a battle between conflicting ideas in our heads, it became more discouraging, expensive, lonely, and difficult. These obstacles may be overcome with patience and careful thought until a therapist is found who feels right. Internalizing erroneous ideas about depression or anxiety—such as, "Just be un-weak!"—made the search to find a therapist harder by causing people to doubt the validity of their feelings. An individual's personal strengths could overcome the obstacles, and feeling a strong connection to a therapist helped to overcome doubts about making such a commitment.

The next chapter examines respondents' feelings and observations about the therapeutic process.

Chapter III

Allowing a Therapeutic Process

> Continuous effort—not strength or intelligence—is the key to unlocking our potential.
>
> Winston Churchill

THERAPY doesn't work by a sprinkling of fairy dust. It entails giving ourselves over to a process in which a remarkable healing power is at work. It happens when we are able to talk about our feelings with someone who listens and understands. We see this in children when they're hurt and need to be comforted; it appears even more reliably when a parent truly listens and allows a child to work out a problem independently. After being genuinely heard, children usually feel soothed and spring back.

Somehow this miracle salve gets lost as we are toughened into adulthood. Emotional wounds often go unattended as hurt gets layered over with admonishments to trudge on, never mind how we might feel. We may be unaware of the ways we numb ourselves to pain yet still protect a sensitive area—until we can't ignore it anymore.

We long to heal when something within us has been lost or broken. Dictionaries describe *therapy* as the treatment of an illness or disability, with a healing power or quality, but it is also a *process* in which the patient moves forward through a series of stages and changes toward a contemplated end. *Psychotherapy* is the treatment of mental and emotional disorders through encouraging communication of conflicts and insight into problems, and in the *process of psychotherapy*, patients give themselves over to whatever feelings and concerns arise in conversation with a therapist, also moving toward an end.

In the process of learning to play a sport or an instrument, you learn to become aware of everything you do and how you do it. In therapy you become more aware of what you say and do, and in the process figure out what you want to change or keep. The idea of a process is important because the goal of therapy is not how fast we complete the course but rather how well we see and understand, how well matters get resolved and wounds healed. Since it's hard to know what success in this endeavor is going to feel like, leaning in to the process is partly an act of faith. It begins with little more than a willingness to talk about those parts of our lives that have become difficult or muddled.

By talking with someone who listens and helps us gain insight into what we came to talk about, healing takes place. It is a connection to another human being. We are trying to talk about what has happened in our lives and how we feel about it. Sometimes it's as if we are being lowered in a bathysphere to a place within us that feels strangely new yet vaguely familiar. Sometimes it's as if with our fingertips, eyes closed, we explore the experience with someone who helps us understand and find the words to explain what we are "seeing." They support us when we feel afraid or feel that we can do no more. By opening ourselves to a greater awareness of our inner life, we begin to heal.

To people outside therapy, as well as to those at work in it, the process seems rather mysterious. In this chapter people tell about their experience of therapy—learning to name feelings, handling other issues that surface, and dealing with doubt. Questions of courage also emerge in this discussion. Does courage have many faces or only one, such as physical courage? Interview participants also talk about aspects of therapy that were uncomfortable or surprising, working through traumatic memories and times when inner stress is expressed physically.

NIMH Comorbidity of Disorders

Comorbidity refers to the co-occurrence of disorders within the same individual. The study determined that 45 percent of those with one mental disorder met criteria for two or more disorders. We have a limited ability to draw clear-cut thresholds beyond which an emotion or behavior becomes a disorder, and boundaries between types of disorders. In addition, severity of mental illness, in terms of disability, is strongly related to comorbidity.[13]

Sarah

Following her brother's suicide and a second failed marriage, Sarah saw three therapists before the one she mentions here. She began to see this one during her developing relationship with Hank.

"My experience with her was very warm. I can just picture coming into her office and she'd say, 'Oh, hi, aren't you gorgeous today,' just real sweet. Her approach was, 'What do you want to talk about?' She's the only one I've been to that was organized. The others were so unorganized it drove me crazy. They never had a plan for me or a goal. It was like this: I'd come in and they'd forget what we talked about a week or two ago, or where we'd leave off, couldn't find my paperwork . . . they weren't ready when I came to sit down. This woman, the first time, said, 'Let's make a goal for you,' and I loved it. We wrote it down, and she helped me through it. It was a feeling that she cared. She wanted to use that hour wisely.

"Talking about things about yourself that you don't want to talk about is hard. Things you don't really want to deal with, things you push down. There's a little bit of embarrassment in the way I think about myself and my life.

"I went into each counselor and knew exactly what I wanted. That was to feel better about myself, increase my self-esteem, learn how to have good relationships with men.

"The first time I was in therapy, I was a little afraid, because it was new. There was a lot of pain with my brother gone and dealing with why he went. And I knew why he did what he did, because he felt the same way I did. That was painful. It was scary because I didn't know where it was going to take me. I had no idea where I was going. I was going through a divorce, and I was trusting her with my life. I just felt I wasn't making the right decisions, wondering if I was thinking straight. I was very confused, and she made me stronger.

"The most difficult issue is, 'Can you really trust this person? Are they really telling you the correct information?' I can't listen to everything she says, because not everything she says is right for me. So I really had to learn in the whole process to pick what I thought would work for me not just because she said so—and that was hard for me to figure out. I didn't feel good about myself, so what she said had to be right. But it wasn't always right.

"Money was always a reason to quit. I would get tired of the counselor. I felt I wasn't going anywhere. It just gets to a point with me, where it's, 'okay, that's it!'

"What surprised me with my first three counselors was that they said, 'You know that your parents killed your brother.' It took me awhile to figure out that they were right. Because of the way my parents are. That was a big surprise. I would never in my dreams have thought of that. I worried about how not normal my childhood was. There was a lack of trust, of emotional love, any kind of affection. It was just all abuse—verbal and emotional. Even my mom was abusive. They both were.

"Weight—up and down—was always a problem for me. I did a lot of stress eating. Depression. For awhile in therapy I had depression as things came out. My asthma and allergies were prime. I was on a lot of medication. The emotional stress had a lot to do with the physical problems."

Feeling Cared About

An aspect of the therapeutic process is whether or not you feel cared about, and this is a fair expectation. Clients will take as evidence different indications that a therapist cares. It might be a willingness to talk about something that annoys you, not changing the appointment time willy-nilly, being able to hang in there through rough patches, or not putting words in your mouth. For Sarah, it was her therapist's organization, willingness to help her set a goal for their work, and dedication to use the hour together wisely. Also, the therapist supported her through feelings of embarrassment, fear, pain, doubt, and confusion. Would Sarah have opened herself to someone who seemed indifferent?

Her goal of improved self-esteem left room for other concerns that came up. Rather than being off the subject, they let her clarify other things that were bothering her. The therapist could see the bigger picture of how one area spilled into another. A nod here, a question there is often enough to let us know they are listening with intent and drawing our attention toward something we may have hurried past. Sarah was surprised to learn about the connection between the conditions of her childhood and her feelings as an adult.

Another concern that surfaced was doubt about her therapist. She may have felt uncomfortable addressing this, but once we enter a therapeutic relationship we have to reckon with our doubts about both the process and the therapist. Perhaps one gauge of the viability of a relationship is whether we can talk about our doubts *about* them *with* them; the good ones will not take offense and will even help us through the discomfort. We can't lean into a process when doubts are buzzing around distracting us, but it is also possible that Sarah's instincts were right about some of the therapists she decided to leave. The answers to our doubts depend in part on the training, sensitivity, and experience of our therapist, and on our willingness and determination to go the distance. We are asked to open ourselves to someone who is trying to help us. Yet sometimes opening those locked chambers may be the most difficult task we ever faced. We need to believe that the person listening won't leave us stranded on the side of the road; we feel cared about when each of our concerns is addressed in a meaningful way.

NIMH Attention Deficit Hyperactivity Disorder (ADHD)

ADHD, one of the most common mental disorders in children and adolescents, also affects an estimated 4.1 percent of adults, ages 18-44, in a given year. ADHD usually becomes evident in preschool or early elementary years. The median age of onset of ADHD is seven years, although the disorder can persist into adolescence and occasionally into adulthood. [14]

Hank

At the time of my interview with Sarah, she and Hank had not yet begun seeing a new therapist for couples' therapy. Several months later when Hank and I talked, he focused largely on their recent sessions with him.

"This guy really caught on quickly as to how we are. He nailed it within forty-five minutes. He said, 'Okay, so when this happens, you react this way or this way.' Exactly! It was like he'd been following us around. He's very upbeat, a likeable guy. Real sharp, real smart. I was very impressed with him right away.

"What's most important to me is how quickly they can understand what we're talking about rather than week after week trying to explain what makes me up, what makes Sarah up, telling the same stories over and over. I like that he caught on real quick. And this guy is not judgmental in any way. You could tell him, 'Oh, I stabbed her in the back,' and he might say, 'Okay, when you were thinking of doing that'. . . He wasn't saying, 'You shouldn't be doing that!' Those are the two biggest things I would look for in someone.

"When I start with a therapist, I always get kind of excited. I go there to solve a problem, so I get excited thinking, 'Okay, we're going to work this out somehow and make something better.' I'm happy to go, happy to start talking about whatever the issues are. Maybe I like talking about myself!" Hank laughs.

"Sometimes the truth hurts. You realize that you're not as perfect as you thought you were. It's humbling. Progress is important to me—it's the only reason to go. You know when you've tapped out with a therapist. You know you've gotten as much as you can, so that's a time when you feel like quitting. Hopefully I won't need to go forever, but I'd like to get some things fixed first. There haven't been any surprises in my therapy, just learning stuff I didn't know.

"I did get frustrated and upset with the second counselor. I can't remember the incident, but a lot of times she made me feel bad about myself. She was harsh. I guess she hurt my feelings. She never intended to, I don't think, but there was one time when I called her up the next day because I couldn't sleep at night after therapy. That was one time that it was pretty bad. A lot of times I walked out of there feeling bad about myself. I guess sometimes the truth hurts, and you don't always like to share that you're not so perfect. There were times that I got upset. But I kept going back.

"My problems have never taken a physical form, other than losing sleep maybe. I don't know that I had any specific goals between Sarah and me. I'd like to see us be a little more tolerant of each other and learn what it takes to be tolerant."

Being Emotionally Engaged

As early as their first meeting, Hank felt their new therapist understood them. The impression was strong, pushing aside the inevitable doubts and concerns. When good feelings accrue at every session, therapist and client are pouring a foundation for their work together.

Hank went to therapy to solve a problem, not because he was falling apart. The harshness of a previous therapist had hurt his feelings so much he couldn't sleep. He called her and left a message. I hoped she felt the strain in their relationship keenly enough to address it at their next meeting.

We can become angry in therapy, and our feelings get hurt, but our trust in the therapist—that we are cared about and won't be hurt—has to be recovered. In my experience, work and progress won't proceed until the breach is mended. Without trust, the intellect moves on without emotional engagement; without it, there is no vulnerability and no change.

Recently I heard a story at a reading workshop for literacy tutors given by a college professor. She told of setting out to mow her lawn, a job her sons usually did, atop a riding lawn mower. After passing a length of the yard she looked back to check her progress and saw the blade mechanism hadn't been engaged. She was moving forward but no grass had been mowed. "It's the same with reading," she said. "The mind has to be engaged when you read."

It's also true in therapy—our emotions have to be engaged along with our intellect or nothing happens. It can take some of us a long time before the blades engage, if ever. The intellect alone doesn't get the job done; emotions and intellect have to work together. Our emotions become engaged when we lower our defenses enough to become vulnerable.

Hank's comments contrast his experiences with three therapists. Without using the words "emotional engagement" and "vulnerability," his meaning is clear. Of the first he said, "There was a real problem, and she wasn't getting to it. I didn't know what the problem was, but I knew she wasn't getting it." Of the second he noted, "She was very harsh in a lot of ways, but she was realistic. What she taught me was that . . . there was really no communication between my wife and myself about feelings." Then Hank describes the first meeting he and Sarah had with the third therapist: "This guy really caught on quickly as to how we are. He nailed it within 45 minutes. . . It was like he'd been following us around." Hank conveys a sense of what it feels like to find a therapist who quickly sees into the heart of a matter.

Hank learned something from each of them, even learning what he didn't like. The third therapist's engagement with them drew them in to the process.

NIMH The Interaction between HIV/AIDS and Aging

Because co-morbidities and HIV may differentially affect certain underserved vulnerable populations (e.g., people with serious mental illness, homeless, prisoners, diverse racial and ethnic groups), the impact of co-morbidities on HIV-related health disparities is an area of importance.[15]

Christine

Christine was not excited about going into therapy. Fortunately her mother recognized the seriousness of bulimia and persuaded her daughter to seek counseling—even making the arrangements through someone at the university where she worked.

Christine recalls early visits with this therapist, whom she saw for awhile in high school. "At the beginning I was scared and nervous. I didn't know what she would think of me. 'What if she thinks I'm crazy? What if she tells me things I'm not going to agree with?' I was nervous that people would find out and think I was crazy. Lots of fear was the main emotion I felt.

"It was hard to admit I had a problem in the first place because I'm such a perfectionist. At first it was difficult talking with somebody about it, because I didn't know her very well. It was a little hard to say what I was thinking. I didn't really want to do it. But then it got really easy, and I didn't have a problem talking to her at all."

Symptoms of bulimia came back when Christine was in college, and she returned to the same therapist.

"Stopping the bulimia was a goal, and I didn't really have any other goals when I was in high school. But when I was in college one of the goals—and I think I articulated this one—was to stop being so shy, to be more outgoing, and be happier, more positive.

"At the beginning, I was afraid. It was mysterious, and I didn't know what was going to happen. But going through it—after the first or second time in high school, when I realized what a nice woman she was, and in college, when I realized she didn't think of me as a failure—I wasn't fearful anymore. It was just uneasiness in the beginning, when I didn't know what would happen.

"In high school, I wanted to quit right away because I thought, 'I get what she's doing! I can do the rest myself now!'" Christine was tearful as she laughed. "I sort of thought I was a little know-it-all, and my mom says, 'I don't think so, Christine.'"

"I kept going, and I'm glad I did because I learned a lot more about myself. I think the reason I wanted to quit was my perfectionism coming out, and I thought, 'I can to do the rest myself now.' But you put it off, and the next thing you know, you haven't done anything, and nothing has changed!

"I was surprised at how the internal dialogues with myself would be so negative. Things that I would never think about other people. The surprise was how I treated myself.

"Something that frustrated me—it wasn't something my therapist did—but she gave me this workbook on self-esteem, and one part was about families and how sometimes families can contribute to low self-esteem or eating disorders. There was a whole chapter on it. I was frustrated with that because I came from a good family! I almost felt like the author of this book was assuming that because I had low self-esteem I came from a dysfunctional family and that upset me. I told my counselor about it the next week, and she said, 'I thought about that afterwards, that that really didn't pertain to you.' But it was nothing that the counselor did.

"My inner problems took a physical form in the bulimia. Also, going along with that, I would exercise too much, like two hours on a treadmill, but no other aches or pains."

Allowing Goals to Evolve

Christine entered therapy the first time with an awareness of one set of feelings, especially fear and wariness. Twice she mentioned a fear of being found out to be crazy. Obviously, she doesn't suffer from severe, debilitating mental illness, so what is that fear about? Perhaps it's about feelings tumbling around in her head that would begin to make sense if she could simply talk about them with someone who understands. Therapy could help her to see that none of her feelings were crazy, though sometimes feelings dress up in bizarre clothes to draw attention to a matter that needs to be worked out.

When she started therapy, fear prevailed. But she found her therapist to be friendly, accepting, and surprisingly easy to talk with. When she returned in college with feelings of failure as the bulimia "resurfaced," she began to see other possibilities for herself ("I learned a lot more about myself"), and began to see how her shyness and low self-esteem were converted to bulimia, an expression of emotional pain. She and her therapist were able to work out a small misunderstanding so they could continue in a productive relationship.

In an environment of trust, rapport, and emotional safety, she was able to talk about her feelings. In high school her goal in therapy was to "stop the bulimia." In college her goals evolved into something larger than just stopping the bulimia; these included being more outgoing and silencing the negative internal conversations.

Allen

Allen describes his experience with a psychologist he consulted about panic attacks. "At the start I felt some fear or reluctance—I'm starting something new. But that was offset by my concerns about becoming housebound. Then other questions came forward: 'Am I going to be compatible with this therapist? Will it be beneficial? Will I be able to work with this person?' I already knew it was important to feel you can work with the therapist.

"It's been difficult to admit to somebody that I'm afflicted with these conditions. Particularly the one that seems so unmanly—of becoming very emotional at times. It was difficult to talk about that initially, but if you're going to get to the bottom of it," he laughed, "you have to be honest and open up about those things. If I cry in front of another man, my thought was, 'If this is going to be helpful, then I have to let it all hang out.' That was difficult at first.

"I was reluctant to discuss things at certain times, but never afraid. I never wanted to quit. I had some questions as to whether we would be able to judge when to end, so we talked about that.

"There were surprises when stuff I learned ran counter to some of the notions I had. The fact that brain functions are tied to chemical reactions was new to me. Physical things and mental things seemed to be separate spheres. I was surprised to learn they are really one sphere.

"I never felt anger during my treatment, but I felt frustration. When I was younger, before the first panic attack occurred, it was exciting to have an opportunity to travel somewhere or be immersed in a situation where you don't know how it will come out. I've not been able to get back to that same feeling. I would like to have gotten back to being unaware of things like panic attacks. But you don't erase that."

Facing Fears

Allen's forthright expression of feeling touched me, even more so because it was difficult to find men who would consent to be interviewed. Many men were in therapy, but few were willing to talk about it. In declining my request, one man said, "You've got to get over the idea that seeing a therapist is about potpourri and doilies"—that is, real men don't go to therapy. Of course that isn't true. But even if we know an idea is absurd, how do we get beyond the idea in our heads? Unlearning is as much a part of the therapeutic process as learning, and it is far, far more difficult. It can entail facing the possibility that we are stupid, weak, worthless, or crazy, so being able to look fear in the face is necessary to the process. Therapy requires enormous courage.

In *Soldier's Heart*, written by a civilian who teaches English literature at West Point, author Elizabeth Samet cites the observation of a sergeant who was diagnosed with depression and posttraumatic stress disorder (PTSD) from a traumatic brain injury in Iraq. It was a story she first heard on National Public Radio. In three months of treatment at Walter Reed, the sergeant realized that—despite heightened awareness of war's devastating psychological impact—the military culture continues to see a higher valor in physical amputees. Meanwhile, "the realm of the mind remains largely invisible." There is an unspoken hierarchy of the wounded. She adds, "[It] echoes our lingering suspicion that psychological wounds are unmanly, something not to be discussed by real warriors."[16]

It's easy to say, "Men shouldn't be embarrassed about being in therapy" just as it is to say, "People with mental illness shouldn't be ashamed." But if you're afraid that maybe you *are* weak (or stupid, cowardly, worthless, etc.), that's a fear you have to face or you won't make yourself vulnerable and won't be emotionally engaged. What makes it possible to get past our fears and faulty beliefs is a good relationship with our therapist. Their belief in us and our trust in them make it possible to do the difficult work of facing our fears; without that, we would be going on a mission with a fellow soldier we don't trust.

If it's true that it's more difficult for men to go into therapy than for women, the irony is inescapable. Allen said he worried that it was unmanly of him to weep over things that touched him, and in the next breath, he said, "If this is going to be helpful, then I have to let it all hang out."

Faces of courage, whether going after the demons within or the enemy in battle, bear up under closer scrutiny. From her students' thoughtful study of literature, Samet writes: "They seemed to understand that courage isn't simply a matter of leading charges: sometimes it consists in speaking up, sometimes in stoic silence, sometimes in forging ahead, sometimes in circumspection, and sometimes in nothing less than preserving our own humanity."[17] And sometimes courage lies in doing something to save one's own life, a kind of moral courage.

As we get to know ourselves in therapy, we have the opportunity to ask questions and to discover answers within ourselves. Knowing ourselves makes us stronger; facing our fears instead of running from them tests then strengthens our courage to face whatever life throws at us.

Nora

Nora's therapy included a chalkboard and concepts. One of these was learning to figure out whether an incident was "real and true" or whether it was a personal, biased interpretation. She had sought help for the relationship with her daughter. "The goals were to get along better with Maureen and maybe to understand myself and figure out what am I doing wrong. Although things still aren't perfect, I am more aware of what works and what doesn't.

"Also, he [her therapist] had asked me a question: 'If I had a concern about my husband, why didn't I confront him?' I thought the therapy was mostly about my daughter, but this came up as well, and he said, 'If this is bothering you, then you need to tell him so and the reason for it. If you guys are so close, why haven't you done this?' That was a good question. That was scary to me, and we finally did talk it over. That was a surprise.

"I wasn't sure about the approach that he was going to take, and I was sort of surprised, because I had never heard of this before. At the beginning, when my answers weren't really where they should have been, I could see where he was coming from and where he was going. So the path was sort of clear. He would map it out. He would draw it out on the chalkboard. It was difficult at first to figure out where he was going. When I was there a little bit, it really wasn't intimidating. All I could think was, 'If this is going to help, I'm for it.' One goal was to understand the concepts, which in turn gave me tools to handle situations. Another goal was to clarify my thinking, so that I would be able to communicate better with my daughter."

Increasing Self-Awareness

We get ourselves into mental ruts, habits of mind we hardly notice. Therapy offers the chance to begin to experience a heightened self-awareness—to ask questions and think about our relationships outside of the ruts. For Nora, an issue surfaced concerning her husband, one that bothered her but that she had let slide. The therapist questioned her. After thinking about it, even though the prospect was scary, she talked the matter over with him and worked it out. In therapy, by increasing awareness of herself and "of what works and what doesn't," she learned to use a set of "tools to handle situations."

She mentions being a little afraid about confronting her husband. Though she doesn't explain why, she nonetheless had to become aware enough of her feelings to recognize the fear, then decide to face it. Her therapist encouraged her and she succeeded. This is not as easy to do as it may appear. We vary considerably in degrees of courage, but a good therapist helps us strengthen that muscle as we become increasingly self-aware and confident in our ability to master things that were formerly impossible.

Greg

Greg saw his elderly mother's therapist and emerged from depression after a relatively brief time in therapy.

"It was up to me to decide what I wanted to talk about. And I didn't know what I wanted to talk about, really. It was kind of uncomfortable at first. There would be long pauses where he would wait for me to say whatever I was thinking. I would have been more comfortable if he had asked a bunch of questions—like a test or something, where you could go down and check off, 'Do you do this?' or 'Do you feel that?' To some extent he guided the conversation, but it was kind of uncomfortable that I had to do almost all the talking, and he didn't say much.

"Then sometimes during the week I'd think, 'Okay, I've got an appointment coming up—What did we talk about last time? Where is this going? Is there something else I can think of that I want to be sure to put on my list to talk about next time?' I didn't have specific goals. It's probably a symptom that when you're depressed you really don't have the energy to get much done. It's hard to tell—even if you have a goal—how close you are to your goal or how much progress you're making.

"It seemed fairly obvious that my depression was related to my mother's Alzheimer's and not some long-ago thing. But I guess there is always a little bit of a fear of 'Okay, what is he going to ask? What's he going to delve into now? Is this related to something more subtle than what it seems like?' There were some of those issues, but I was pretty open with him if he did ask some question about my childhood.

"I was a little surprised that it was so open-ended, that it was up to me to start the conversation, talk about whatever I wanted to talk about. I didn't know what I should be talking about—I'm kind of expecting him to take a more direct approach or ask questions. So that surprised me. With this, more of it was on me than in a normal MD relationship."

Tolerating Therapy's Discomforts

Greg frankly describes the discomfort of unstructured sessions with his therapist and the anxiety of wondering where the conversation and questions might lead. There may have been more to talk about, but Greg didn't seem to need or want it. He soon resumed his life with a greater measure of understanding and acceptance of his mother's condition.

We see a therapist when we can't shake off a depression or work out a problem by ourselves. We can't seem to crack the code, as if surely there must be one. Human nature wants to keep at arm's length whatever we don't want to know, feelings we don't want to feel. Sometimes these tendencies cause people to quit therapy because they so fervently don't want to know or remember. Sometimes the misery needs to be great enough to keep us in treatment but not so great that we can't bear it; this requires great skill and sensitivity in a therapist.

For those who remain in treatment to work through the discomfort, bringing these feelings and patterns of response into awareness greatly eases their burden.

James

Following his partner's accident, James had already established a relationship with the therapist they saw together, but now he wanted to talk just about his concerns.

"At first it felt that there was a whole lot bottled up—a flood of emotion that I wanted to get out, yet I couldn't say the first word. I don't remember exactly how, but he would just get me talking. I looked forward to going and found it empowering. The difficult time was outside of therapy, realizing that I was headed towards something very unpleasant—a decision that I was going to make. To let go of my partner without abandoning him. That was difficult.

"One of my goals was to move ahead with my life without guilt or regret. Definitely I felt afraid. I was looking forward to the change, but I was also afraid. I spent the first year trying to convince my therapist and myself that I was doing okay. Trying to 'look healthy' and reasonable, coping well, etc. In the back of my mind I felt a need to impress him with my insights and healthy assessment of my life. It became clear over time that I wasn't being as honest as I could with myself, or him.

"I was surprised at how little it seemed the therapist did and said but how much he actually did do and say, through my own process. I thought there would be more interchange, more energy, more dialogue, more emotion between the therapist and me. And it was very much not like that. It was all me.

"Also, I remember feeling, 'Here I am again, saying the same things, and nothing has changed.' I would feel angry that there hadn't been more progress. I was embarrassed that I was continuing to do the same things yet expecting different results. And because no one was pushing me—including my therapist—it took me time to realize that I am doing the same thing over and over again and I need to change! The anger was that it wasn't happening quickly enough."

Allowing Enough Time

James alludes to the quiet of the therapeutic space as he rides out the see saw pattern of having a lot to say and nothing to say. We hear him as he begins to hear himself think and wonder aloud, with the therapist's listening presence as support: "It was all me."

He was also angry, frustrated, and embarrassed by what seemed a lack of progress as he kept doing the same things "yet expecting different results." The crucial phrase, "it took me time to realize," is precisely the point. Our thinking goes in mental ruts. We'd far rather the therapist would give us "the answer" so we could get beyond the discomfort. But it is not the therapist's answer that will bring about change and growth. It is coming to it ourselves, and sometimes this takes more time than we'd like. We grow by doing things ourselves rather than having them done for us. It takes time to gain the footing needed to go forward, to find courage, and to ascertain unwelcome truths.

NIMH "Medical Prisoners of War"

Fewer than one percent of Americans have served in Iraq or Afghanistan - 2.7 million men and women over this past decade. Most were under 25, many had never traveled before, and all were volunteers. Over 5,000 died in combat. For many more, war has meant so called "invisible wounds": the improvement in body armor has protected limbs and lives, but not brains and minds. Since the beginning of these wars in 2003, there have been at least 126,000 cases of traumatic brain injury and 70,000 cases of PTSD. At the One Mind meeting, Patrick Kennedy, stressing the urgency of these injuries, called these soldiers "medical prisoners of war."[18]

Claire

Claire took an overdose of pills, saw a therapist for six months, and then resumed her life without therapy. After a few years and "a lot of disastrous relationships with men," she fell into a depression that caused her to seek professional help.

"The first experience after the overdose was just sitting and talking and getting something back from the therapist. In the second experience, I thought it was going to be the same—just sit down and have a nice talk. Something intellectual. But I was quickly dissuaded of that idea. To deal with some of my problems, I had to get in touch with my feelings. I'm not sure I can explain how that happened, but it involved getting very uncomfortable at times. That was what I hadn't reckoned for in therapy. I just thought I'd sit and talk to somebody and talk about the things that were wrong with me.

You know, 'Tell me why these things in my life are wrong!' Claire laughs. "He did give me feedback sometimes, but it was more a process of self-discovery.

"I grew up not understanding what boundaries were. I didn't know that I had the right to say no to people. If somebody asked me to do something, that extended to a lot of areas of my life—to work, to social situations, certainly to sexual relationships with men—and because I had been so enmeshed with my mother, I hadn't learned to build boundaries. I didn't see myself as a separate person from my mother. Over the years he [therapist] taught me to have good boundaries and to say no when I wanted to say no. As I learned more about who I was, I was able to do that.

"What I do remember is that the first few therapy sessions that I went in, he kept asking me the same question in therapy, and that was, 'What do you want?' And I sat there and couldn't answer because I had never thought about what I wanted. In fact, I could hardly speak at all for the first few sessions."

Then she added, "Therapy is an incredible journey that doesn't end, even when you stop going."

Learning to Name Feelings

Claire tells how she had to learn to get in touch with her feelings, which involved "getting very uncomfortable at times." She thought therapy would be having a nice chat, an exchange of pleasantries, getting information and answers. It turned out to be a process of self-discovery, again with the therapist providing feedback and support.

Elementary as it sounds, in therapy we may learn to recognize and name our feelings; we learn to listen for them. Some of us grow up in families where the expression of feelings is discouraged or even punished. It's possible then to become disconnected from a vital part of ourselves, unable to connect with others, or to know what we like or want. We become a good sport or a good soldier, unequipped to deal with our emotions or those of others.

For example, we may not recognize subtle feelings of anxiety or a habit of disregarding them. Therapy may heighten awareness not only of the feeling itself but possibly of the subtle ways anxiety directs some of the choices we make. Our therapist may help us trace the origin of these feelings or help us untangle the threads of our lives by carefully separating one feeling from others to see where it leads. We may not admit how angry we are with someone or about something that happened to us or the ways that anger infects our lives. That's what I mean by "learning to name feelings."

Naming and knowing our feelings, being in touch with and recognizing them, are paths to becoming well. Like people who speak the language of music, who detect subtle differences in chords and harmonies, in therapy we may learn to become more fluent in the language of our emotional life. As with any language, some become highly skilled; others of us learn at least enough to get around in the world more easily. Claire described what she learned in therapy as a journey that didn't end, even when she stopped going. She became more attuned to her inner life.

Rose

"I have felt in conflict with staying in therapy because it would get so rough that every few minutes I was quitting. He's [therapist] always said that it is a work against resistance. One doesn't go in there and just willingly spill your guts. One resists it at every turn in the road because that's what we've been doing all our lives.

"I still don't let myself spend the time crying, and it's a real issue because I don't have outpourings. I don't get rid of the grief. I make up ways to keep it. But I'm working on it.

"There were times when I was there six times a week, because things get very fragile. There has to be a strong sense of protection, otherwise you can't go there. Now, I'm talking as a layman who went through it, but whatever was being brought up because of this intense, on-the-couch, deep analysis led to a lot of fears. And I do remember my therapist saying to me very often, 'Nothing bad is happening now.' But it doesn't feel that way. It feels like it's happening *now*. Because whatever you're remembering—whatever got you to the point that you needed to be in this kind of treatment—is coming to the fore. Sure you feel fear, but the strength of the relationship carries you through that fear.

"If you're delving into your psyche and you don't have surprises, it would be a surprise! The reason you're doing all this is to find out stuff you don't know you know. The insight, the surprises, are the most important part of it. You don't always get there, but there are a lot of surprises.

"The major one for me, probably the hardest one, was when I realized I had no sense of self. I don't remember how at the time I thought about it, but I would say 'egoless.' I just felt like I was everybody's rag doll. I remember being aware that I had no core. That was a surprise, because I always thought I was pretty strong growing up. My image of myself and what I told the rest of the world was that I was a happy and secure kid, I grew up in a nice house, and so on. To think that I didn't have a core was shocking to me. In some ways, that was probably the biggest surprise, because it was so unexpected. To think that I felt like I was nothing, when here I thought I was everything! That was tough.

"Initially my physical health was better. I was always getting colds and feeling miserable, and when I first started therapy, a lot of that went away. But I go through all kinds of physical manifestations of an emotional problem that is easier for me to show physically than emotionally. I don't cry, and I don't get angry easily there, so it comes out in other ways."

Accepting Our Avoidance of Issues

Rose describes how being in therapy was so rough at times she was "quitting every few minutes." No one, she added, goes in there and spills their guts. "One resists it at every turn in the road because that's what we've been doing all our lives." Not wanting to know or remember is what caused the trouble in the first place.

Avoiding issues is "normal," but the effect of continued avoidance takes a toll whether we admit it or not, whether we see it or not. The wish to flee is not surprising, nor is the fact that the only reason any of us can continue the work is because of the relationship with our therapist.

In therapy that goes beneath the surface to unearth what is buried there, the process becomes so intense that the urge to quit can overpower the wish to become well. No one wants to re-experience the pain. Those who have sustained losses and other trauma may need help finding the grief and expressing the anger that should have accompanied the experience. Instead, bottled-up grief may be expressed in physical illness, an excessive need for control, or even premature death.

Rose and others here allude to the ways their bodies express feelings that lie beneath the surface of their awareness. They protect themselves from the knowledge of the difficult experiences, comfort themselves with revised versions of events, or simply "forget" what happened—but the body remembers and expresses the pain.

Because of the stigma of emotional problems and the ease of solving obvious "physical" problems with medication, too little of the information about therapy reaches public awareness. Needless to say, it is expensive and futile to treat only the symptoms and not the underlying cause of illness. In the process of therapy, people strive to uproot the sources of their unease (and "dis-ease") even though fully half the time they exert tremendous effort to avoid the issue they came to deal with, often leaving before they see it through. Being aware of this tendency—it is true of *all* of us—may help you decide to keep trying to stand up to what you most dread; such triumphs are quiet and everlasting.

NIMH Half the Cases of Mental Illness Begin Early

Research shows that half of all lifetime cases of mental illness begin by age 14. Scientists are discovering that changes in the body leading to mental illness may start much earlier, before any symptoms appear. Through greater understanding of when and how fast specific areas of children's brains develop, we are learning more about the early stages of a wide range of mental illnesses that appear later in life...Once mental illness develops, it becomes a regular part of your child's behavior and more difficult to treat. Even though we know how to treat (though not yet cure) many disorders, many children with mental illnesses are not getting treatment.[19]

Jenny

In the course of treatment, Jenny began to see the extent of the emotional, physical, and sexual abuses she suffered in her family.

"When I began therapy, I was scared. I've always known that I was sexually abused, but I didn't know my mom's component, and I didn't have any sense of the extent or the severity of the abuse. With my first therapist, I was not aware of these things, and so I was always afraid, but I didn't know what I was afraid of. I felt very frustrated because he couldn't help me.

"But fear was the biggest thing—of being vulnerable, of all those bad things, which were replaying in the back of my mind, of experiencing those things again. It hurts, but I've never had a session where I experienced something that I didn't leave there feeling so much better after purging this stuff.

"Have I found anything difficult in therapy?" Jenny laughs. "It would be easier to ask what haven't I found difficult!" She laughs again. "Facing myself every day, facing myself in therapy. Trusting. Laying myself open to let someone else know those bad things about me. Fear keeps me from a lot of things as far as success in career and stuff and might keep me from success in friendships, but it doesn't keep me from continuing in therapy.

"The biggest surprise in therapy was when I first remembered my mother sexually abusing me. That was huge. Another shock was when I remembered my stepfather forcing his penis down my throat. Because that was the first time I realized that it went beyond fondling. I had always remembered fondling. And violence in our home. But I couldn't remember much of anything for many, many years.

"I feel like I've got more than a lifetime of pain and being screwed up to come through. I don't have any problem with the amount of time I've been in therapy. If it's the same again as much, I don't have any problem with that. What are my options? I can either quit—which would leave me not finished, and not to my full potential as a person, as a mom—or I can keep putting one foot in front of the other till I reach a point where I feel good about myself more often than not."

Working Through Traumatic Memories

To feel some peace, those who have experienced severe trauma must work through their memories and recover the feelings about what happened. After a tough session during which the traumatic experiences are relived, when feelings return full force, exhaustion and relief roll in. Jenny described it as "feeling so much better after purging this stuff."

Her story is filled with courage, but after "purging" there is more work to do. Feeling relief is only part of the therapeutic hurdle. We have to be able to talk about it, keep returning to the events and giving words to our memories until they are drained of their power over us.

In *Trauma and Recovery*, Judith Herman writes, "It is understandable for both patient and therapist to wish for a magic transformation, a purging of the evil of the trauma. Psychotherapy, however, does not get rid of the trauma. The goal of recounting the trauma story is integration, not exorcism. In the process of reconstruction, the trauma story does undergo a transformation, but only in the sense of becoming more present and more real. The fundamental premise of the psychotherapeutic work is a belief in the restorative power of truth-telling."[20]

Achieving mastery can take years of work. When we can talk about it without feeling sick or crying, trembling or flinching, shaking, retreating, or shutting down, when we can gaze coldly and sadly at what happened, it has become fully part of our knowledge of ourselves. The memory of what happened is no longer searing, no longer seizes us by the throat.

Not everyone who chooses open-ended therapy is there because of a history of maltreatment or abuse. Some do it because they want a deeper understanding of themselves. Or, they may feel their creative potential blocked and suspect they are being constrained by something within themselves.

Beth makes the point that not everyone *wants* to know themselves better, but she does.

NIMH Effects of Abuse

Adults who were physically abused, sexually abused, or severely neglected as children were significantly more likely to be unemployed, living below the poverty line, and using social services than people without a history of childhood maltreatment. Having experienced more than one type of maltreatment increased these risks further. Overall, adults who had experienced any type of maltreatment in childhood were twice as likely as non-victims to be unemployed. Childhood physical abuse and a history of multiple types of maltreatment accounted for this trend, increasing risk of unemployment by 140 percent and 190 percent, respectively.[21]

Beth

Beth found a way to end her first treatment relationship when the therapist kept nodding off. Even though Beth took offense when her therapist was not fully engaged in the work, she felt overall the therapy had helped her.

Years later she has found a new therapist. Again she felt nervous about what she would learn, but also excited. At times she feels shame, hurt, embarrassed, and afraid—all difficult—but she wants to understand why she continues to feel bad about herself, including what part she plays in continuing to have those bad feelings.

"I'm afraid of talking about certain family-of-origin things that I want to learn more about—but I don't want to learn more about. In my first therapy, I wanted to quit when the nodding off would start, but I was too embarrassed. If that happened now, I would handle it differently. I would say something about it instead of blaming myself, and that's huge growth." She goes on to say that it surprises her, yet it doesn't, that she is so sensitive to her new therapist's response to her, that even a minute slight can be painful.

"I don't have any qualms about 'It's taking so long,' or 'It's going so slow.' We as human beings—me as an individual—are very complicated. I'm trying to look at parts of my life that go back for as long as I can remember. It makes sense that we kind of meander about whatever comes up."

As she prepares to change to twice weekly sessions, instead of once a week, she admits the shift is hard. "Not because it means I am more 'crazy,' but because I will be more dependent. I don't want that because 'If I don't depend on you, you can't hurt me.' It has a lot of meaning to it that I have yet to understand."

This became the rare instance in which I stepped out of the list of questions I asked each person. I was curious about the route Beth had taken by choosing to get her doctorate in a psychodevelopmentally oriented therapy. This open-ended type of therapy is not everyone's choice, and certainly not possible for everyone, but our conversation was an opportunity to learn something I wanted to know. Thus, before we wrapped up our first meeting, I asked her to reflect on some of the influences that caused her to adopt this approach to therapy.

She explained that her first job as a social worker was in a residential treatment center working with traumatized children.

"I had a variety of workbooks and therapeutic games that were of the cognitive behavioral type. I had my armor, so to speak, of all these ideas. And, boy, did they flop. They just flopped! Every once in awhile some worksheet that I tried or some game was helpful—but that was the exception.

"In that setting I was working with 'How do I get a person in the room with me?' Sometimes literally in the room with me, but also emotionally in the room with me. It didn't matter what catchy little cognitive behavioral piece I had, if that trust and connection, that sense of safety—not even connection!—wasn't there.

"These children feared me as they did any other person in their life because they had been so maltreated. A lot of these kids' experiences were such that they didn't know me from anybody. And the 'anybodies' they did know caused them great harm. Why would they think that I wouldn't hurt them?

"That was what I was up against. How to help kids *be* with me. That became the whole therapy. That became the year's worth of work! How the child and I handle that. So, some cognitive behavioral approaches might have been helpful at times, but they never really addressed *that* piece. And without that, how can any work even begin?

"That was probably my first conscious experience of really looking at what was going on in the treatment relationship. Prior to that I was always interested in people and why they do what they do and what meanings people give to various experiences. This person does this and this person does that—what's that all about? I was aware and interested, but as it played out in the treatment relationships, these were my first experiences that put me smack dab in the middle of 'How do I do this?'

"I didn't throw out all those worksheets. They're helpful in different settings. Initially, I thought of them as tools to fall back on. I thought, 'If we can just help them manage their thoughts, or change their thoughts, or change their behavior, it's going to make a difference.' And it didn't.

"When I think of a psychodynamic therapy, it acknowledges the power of the unconscious as being a significant motivator in human behavior. That we do things for reasons that we're aware of, but also not aware of. At times, humans can be extremely contradictory—on the one hand, because of what they're thinking, but on the other hand, because of reasons that are influencing them that they're not fully aware of.

"It takes a look at past experiences, past relationships, and how those relationships have shaped us to be the person we are, how they're still alive in us, how we seek familiarity in our relationships. Maybe we consciously or unconsciously continue the same way of relating, or the same experience of being related to, without being fully aware of that.

"It takes into consideration the treatment relationship and the patient's hopes, wishes, fears, dread, longings about the therapist in particular, based on their past relationships with significant others. That behavior has several meanings to it, and we are shaped from infancy."

Recognizing Achievements

Sometimes all we want of a therapist is a safe harbor. Once this is secured our goals may shift. We may want to make good use of the chance to learn more and grow. Once the work of therapy has begun, we also want to feel we are making progress *toward a contemplated end.* Achievements are usually subtle, without ceremony or fanfare. Certificates are not issued because the experience is internal, such as a different way of looking at or handling a situation. Beth said of her first therapist who would nod off, "If that happened now, I would handle it differently. I would say something about it instead of blaming myself, and that's huge growth." She recognizes her achievement.

Now with a new therapist she sees herself advancing and wants more. But with the prospect of seeing her therapist twice a week looms the idea of becoming more dependent. She finds this distressing, wonders why, then decides, "'If I don't depend on you, you can't hurt me.' It has a lot of meaning to it that I have yet to understand."

Beth doesn't yet know what it means, but it means something and she intends to find out. By becoming more self-aware, where we notice more about how we feel and react, we observe changes to our thinking and to ways we handle situations. These quiet achievements are what we're after. They have a long reach into our lives, and without them we stay in the same rut of whatever it is that causes us, for example, to pull back, perhaps from closeness or from success, throw up a wall, or shut down.

What I recognize in Beth's comments is that forward-and-back aspect of therapy's searching process: "I want to know, but I don't want to know; I want to get better, but sometimes I don't; I want to change, but I would rather stay the same." Therapy is not a rocket trip into a better life. If allowed to meander, related issues surface to offer both client and therapist a clearer picture. Clarity leads to a more complete understanding and resolution of issues that interfere in a person's life.

As I read Beth's comments again, I also recognize the reaching, as if into inner darkness, to understand why being dependent on her therapist feels so uncomfortable and why feelings about herself seem to have no rational explanation. She says, "I want to find out why I feel so bad about myself, and why I'm continuing to torture myself—if I say I don't want to feel bad anymore! Darn it! Why do I seem to keep doing it? What part am I playing in that process?"

Asking the question, "What part am I playing in that process?" means being able to tolerate pools of self-doubt and to look closely at ways she contributes to her unease. Beth's questions are not trivial. Once the code is cracked, her relief from these feelings will trickle into all the crevices of her life.

We seem to be observing Beth's awareness of herself unfold. It is as if she knew things about herself, yet didn't know them (or didn't want to know them), and in a supportive therapeutic relationship she is coming to understand and accept these and other aspects of herself. With a recognition of how complex she is as an individual, she is realistic about the time and money involved in knowing herself more deeply—though not without some resentment on both counts.

NIMH Substance Abuse May Co-Exist with Depression

Alcohol and other substance abuse or dependence may also co-exist with depression. Research shows that mood disorders and substance abuse commonly occur together.[22]

Summing Up

In a therapeutic process we give ourselves over to whatever feelings and concerns arise with a therapist whom we see for help in sorting out something that weighs heavily on us or has plagued us for a long time. The idea is to shift our focus—understandable, but misguided—from how fast we can accomplish our goal to one in which we allow thoughts and feelings to meander, not trying to control the process too much, letting concerns surface gradually.

Unlike examples of other successes, few people share the importance of therapy in their lives or the effort it took to achieve relief from their troubles. Leaning in to such a process is an act of faith, especially since it is hard to know what success in this endeavor is going to feel like. It begins simply with a willingness to talk about those parts of our lives that have become difficult and to wonder why.

This chapter used participants' comments about the therapeutic process to illustrate aspects of therapy that contributed to a satisfactory outcome. We saw reasons for learning to name feelings and the irony of wanting to get better, yet fighting the process tooth and nail. We saw some of therapy's surprises. We considered the pain and fear of facing ourselves, and the nature of courage, especially in relation to men and women in the military culture.

As in previous chapters, we looked at both situational and open-ended therapies, and the matter of time. Aspects of working through traumatic memories were explored, along with reasons in favor of staying in treatment.

In the next chapter, interview participants take a longer view of issues related to their therapy. I've called these "afterthoughts," by which I mean assessing therapy's impact on our lives whether we have ended treatment, are taking a break from it, or continue working. My respondents talk about the struggle of remaining in treatment, stigma, and the rewards of working through emotional problems to a clearer finish. Also we explore such themes as the emotional education therapy bestows and thoughts about what therapy hasn't cured.

Chapter IV

Afterthoughts about Therapy

Courage is resistance to fear, mastery of fear, not absence of fear.
Mark Twain

A PIANO has ten thousand parts to bring into tune. Imagine how much more complex it is to bring a person, through therapy, "into tune"—nor can such delicate work be accomplished in a mere hour or two.

Ideas about therapy are one thing when we are in its midst, but viewing it from a distance, when we have a body of experience to draw on, offers a complementary perspective. In a similar vein, the first-time parent of a newborn has one perspective about the experience and another by the time the child turns two. This chapter explores therapy's effect on my respondents' lives to see what has changed after the passing of time, whether they have continued in treatment or not. My questions addressed the difficulty of remaining in treatment (if any, aside from time and money), awareness of stigma, feelings about what was left "uncured," and personal qualities that contributed to a good outcome.

Therapists ask questions that nudge us to reflect on our feelings and experiences. Our replies often lead the conversation elsewhere. So it was with the questions I asked of interview participants—not just their answers were interesting, but also the surprising places where their reflections sometimes led.

As they thought about their experiences, several ideas came forth. One was the idea of therapy as an education; the idea of accountability; of being afraid to admit to a problem. One interviewee describes looking for herself in books, another tells of her tendency to intellectualize rather than feel, and another about no longer holding onto a "distorted, hurtful version" of herself.

Sarah

Sarah had entered therapy following her brother's suicide. She saw several counselors as she tried to come to terms with her feelings about his death. She began especially to think about their family. As her second marriage dissolved, she continued with another therapist, trying to understand what had drawn her to another ill-fated relationship. As these issues were sorted out and her confidence improved, she met Hank. They have worked in therapy individually and as a couple to forge a better relationship than either of them previously had.

"Time and money make it difficult to remain in treatment. Sometimes I didn't feel like dealing with my crap. It was too emotionally wearing. It's like anything else: you have to just keep going. You have to just plow through it. It wasn't easy.

"I've needed therapy because of my childhood. It's not something I can explain. It's just something you know inside of you that isn't right. You know you're feeling this way, but you also know you shouldn't be. It's not like someone had to tell me to go. Something was always there that I knew I needed to go.

"I don't know why I was open to getting help. They would say in an alcoholic family there's always a strong child who is determined. Maybe that was me. I was always determined to make myself better. I got tired of feeling the way I did.

"Books were helpful, especially books about children of alcoholics. I was intrigued by them. I would think, 'Wow, someone else felt like this, too? It's not just me.' One woman wrote about how she felt about herself and her sexuality. To this day when I see my dad I worry about what I wear. I don't know. It's weird. It's a weird relationship. I feel uncomfortable. I tend to cover myself more around my dad. I have a sense of disapproval and shame.

"There's a lot that therapy hasn't 'cured,' such as my insecurity in a relationship. Trusting a man completely. I'm better at it, but I still can't seem to find that therapist that can really get inside and understand it. I think my counselors have tended to look at me and say, 'But why?' They just seem to think it's so easy to cure, and it's not. I really struggle with that. I don't think it will work out in time because it's been a long time. It could if I found the right therapist. But I wouldn't even know how to go about finding the right one, spending a lot of money, and going through my entire life story—which would drive me crazy."

Sarah knew felt her childhood lacked sufficient support to help her become more self-confident and secure in her relationships. Although therapy helped, she felt she would need more to bring the peace she longed for.

Searching for Peace

Sarah's comment, "I got tired of feeling the way I did," was an impetus for going to therapy. Though she is doing better—sometimes much better—she seems to have a deepening awareness of her family's insufficiencies and her ongoing struggle with insecurity in a relationship. A few notes of frustration, longing, and weariness sound in her voice, even on the page.

Not everyone is interested in an open-ended, insight-oriented therapy. For most people, time and money are limited. But being tired of feeling the same way over a long period of time can be a reason for trying therapy again, one that may be less solution-focused, one where you explore issues of the family and the origin of your own puzzling feelings. I like to think this smorgasbord of others' experiences in therapy may give you, the reader, some idea of possibilities and offer the encouragement to see it through. Therapy is one way of being able to find a measure of peace, and more often than we could know, a great deal more.

NIMH Mental Disorders Commonly Start Early in Life

About 20 percent of U.S. youth during their lifetime are affected by some type of mental disorder to an extent that they have difficulty functioning...The data support the observation from surveys of adults that mental disorders most commonly start in early life.[23]

Hank

Hank and his first wife went into counseling hoping to save their marriage. He felt his wife simmered with a low-level anger. Frustrated by the lack of communication, even with counseling, Hank and his wife divorced. When he met Sarah, they agreed on the importance of working together with a new counselor on issues they identified early in their developing relationship, then again with another therapist after they had lived together a few years.

"I wouldn't say it's ever been difficult to remain in therapy . . . once I realized I'd gotten as much out of the person as I could, there was no point in coming anymore.

"Initially, if there are issues between people, you need to resolve them. Sometimes you need therapy to find out how. There are some very narrow-minded people where I work, who'd say, 'That's not what I'd do! I'd go have a beer!' I think because I'm more educated than that in terms of therapy, I realize by that education that it's nothing to be ashamed of.

"My mom had seen a counselor when I was a kid, and I feel it helped her a lot. My mom and dad had some marital problems and it tore up the family pretty bad, but they worked it out. It was mainly because my mom got help and realized why my dad was doing the things he was doing, and what she could do . . . I believe if she hadn't gotten help they probably wouldn't have stayed together.

"I would say that I probably take things still too personally, which I shouldn't. I know probably ninety percent of the things that happen aren't because of me personally—but it's hard not to take it personally. That's a tough one, and I need to still learn that. It might work out in time if I keep beating it into my brain, 'It's not personal!'"

Becoming Educated by Therapy

Hank's comment hit me: "I'm more educated than that in terms of therapy." Therapy itself educates us in ways that we don't find in textbooks, ways that help to resolve difficult issues. The idea that therapy "educates" us implies a lasting change in our thinking and perception. When it happens, there is no need to "keep beating" anything into anyone's brain because something has been *resolved* and we are more at peace about it.

Many people, including some therapists, are "well educated" in terms of academic degrees, but their lives may be emotionally impaired. Perhaps because of their success in other areas, they see no need for therapy; or like the rest of us, they don't want to face their stuff. It's easy for the intellect, especially if it's a very good one, to assume superiority. But progress in therapy draws its strength from a different source than intellect alone. It can be hard to put aside a reliance on intellectual achievement and open oneself to another person. Emotional limitations may not interfere with intellectual achievement, but it can allow tangible gains to substitute for deeper emotional capacities. I think of parents who are caught up in career strivings and then are surprised when one of their children begins to show signs of stress or even depression.

But, like a muscle, our emotional lives can be enlarged. Some of us who did not learn from our families how to resolve differences with others can learn how in therapy. Having a college degree, even several of them, does not bestow this knowledge, nor is it where we learn how to love. If not in our families, or in an exceptional friendship, then in therapy we can learn how it feels when an issue is resolved and when it isn't. We can *learn* how to discern that. Once we learn how with our therapist, that ability is transferred to other relationships and to helping our children learn how.

People can succeed in this endeavor and deepen their relationships without advanced degrees, wealth, or family connections. Instead, therapy asks for an open mind, a willing heart, and—my therapist tells me—hope.

Therapy's potential to educate us about our very human interactions deserves wider publicity. In therapy, Hank learned a few things that helped him in relationships with Sarah and his daughter—especially how to talk with each other about their feelings.

The amicable relationship with his former wife gives their daughter a climate in which to grow that is without rancor as she shuttles between the two parents she loves. A bitter relationship after divorce, marked by vindictive acts and manipulations, hurts children. In a culture where divorce is so common, one potential benefit of therapy is to help willing parties put their anger into words in the therapist's office instead of unleashing it on their hapless children or acting it out on a family stage with their children as witnesses to bitter strife.

Instead of turning away those persistently uncomfortable feelings—having a beer is one way—therapy helps us look beneath the surface to understand our feelings in the context of a situation. The education we receive in our emotional life (and that of others) deepens our range of tolerance for complexity and ambiguity, helps us withhold judgment and look more deeply into a set of circumstances. Through it we can extend our emotional range and capacity for empathy. Universities don't yet offer such possibilities.

Christine

Christine described how afraid she was of going to see a therapist for the first time while in high school. She feared she would learn she was crazy or that her friends would find out she was in therapy. Even though she wanted to put an end to the bulimia, at the same time she didn't want to admit she had a problem. She felt much more at ease with her counselor after one or two visits, but not without wanting to quit to be her own therapist. Her mother's comment, "I don't think so, Christine," helped her stay in therapy until she had learned more about herself to bring some of bulimia's symptoms under better control.

"In high school, at the beginning, I thought I could do it myself. But when in therapy we started delving deeper into my problems, I realized I wouldn't be able to fix it myself. I had very supportive parents, which helped a lot." Without support from them, Christine's work in therapy would have been more difficult.

"I realized all the serious physical problems that can come with bulimia, and that scared me into going as well. Realizing that I couldn't do it myself helped me to go.

"There are still times when I'll need to purge. I'll feel guilty after eating, but I'm a lot better and it's something I'm working on. It's not something you cure immediately. People deal with it for years and years.

"This time I'm more optimistic. I'm more mature and I realize more the *reasons* why I've done things, and I can catch myself, so I think eventually . . . it will take awhile, but I think I will get completely better." Christine becomes tearful, saying, "I cry really easily!" then laughs and adds, "I'm fine!"

"My therapist gave me a self-esteem workbook. At first I thought it would be sort of silly, but it made me write things down. I had to make concrete what I was thinking. It wasn't some vague notion. That helped me realize what I was feeling. Putting my feelings into words.

"Once I got past the stigma, I was open-minded about it. It wasn't set in stone that I would never go. Maybe being persistent, being a perfectionist, helped too. It has its good points," she laughs. "I wanted to get this licked.

Intelligence. Diligence. Doing the work, even after going to the therapist, not just forgetting about it till the next session—a good work ethic."

Being Held to Account

The wish to "do it myself" was such a common theme from many people I spoke with that I came to feel it was healthy—a wish to be independent rather than dependent. But only to a point. For all of these people, a decision prevailed in favor of therapy, whether their own or that of someone who cared about them and who saw the need for professional help. That struggle between opposing forces was intense—one voice telling us we could (or should) do it ourselves and the other saying, "Maybe getting some help is not a bad idea."

As opposed to the do-it-yourself approach she preferred, Christine made several comments about the value of seeing a therapist that seem especially wise. The appointment with the therapist holds us accountable because we return to face the issue rather than ducking it. Furthermore, seeking to understand us—and to help us understand ourselves—the therapist asks questions that cause us to consider a point from different angles. We find ourselves thinking intently about something today that only yesterday we took for granted or didn't see at all. Also, we make our feelings "concrete" by saying or writing them, especially those we share with our therapist.

A commonly held belief is that we can do it ourselves without submitting to the therapeutic process. Even after entering therapy, this idea often persists. It is as if we must outwit our therapist, prove who is smarter, or convince her or him of how much we don't need to be here, instead of leaning into and finding strength in the relationship. We may learn in time that this strength carries over to strength within ourselves and to closer relationships with others. Many of us would have retreated further and further from life were it not for the relationship we have with our therapist.

Conversations with a caring therapist hold us accountable by helping us face what we most want to avoid. By facing ourselves, we are strengthened to face the world anew.

NIMH Mental Disorders in Youth

Overall, nearly half of the sample reported having met diagnostic

> criteria for at least one disorder over a lifetime, and about 20 percent reported that they suffered from a mental disorder with symptoms severe enough to impair their daily lives... The researchers also noted strong links between parental characteristics and their teen's disorders. For example, children of parents with less education (e.g., no college degree) were at an increased risk for having any kind of mental disorder. And compared to teens with married or cohabiting parents, those with divorced parents also were at higher risk for a disorder, especially anxiety, behavior and substance use disorders.[24]

Greg

I asked Greg if he read about depression before or during his experience of it. He had a ready answer. "Reading can help you get in the right mind set, and maybe do some of the background research, but the therapist is not just some amateur. He's not just a good friend you would do this with. This is a trained person who has dealt with this before and knows how to do it. With a lot of things, you really need to take the class. You don't just read the book and learn calculus. You need to have the trained instructor."

Needing to Take the Class

A commonly held belief is that we can do it ourselves without submitting to the therapeutic process; just read about it. Even after entering therapy, this idea often rides shotgun. It is as if we must prove to the therapist that we already know this stuff, instead of allowing ourselves to explore various sides of a situation that confronts us. Reading about psychology, yet never summoning the courage to go into therapy, is like reading about sex, a trip to the Rocky Mountains, or how to create a perfect omelette. It's not the same as the experience itself. Merely reading about it may be another form of avoidance (fear of what you will learn about yourself), one that might prove worth taking a closer look.

Allen

Allen tried on his own, without success, to undo the tightening grip of panic attacks. For years he attempted to work out his problems without the help of a therapist. Once he got help, he began to learn a lot about his panic attacks. Important in managing them was the realization that "physical things" and "mental things" are not separate spheres, but one and the same. He brought an explorer's spirit to therapy. Having been cautioned that issues under discussion can take time to resolve, he drew on patience as an ally, worked through discomfort, and faced his issues squarely.

"I entered therapy because I couldn't come to a solution on my own. I needed the help of people who are trained in these areas—I just couldn't do it on my own. And I tried!" he laughs. "I had worked at doing it on my own, trying to touch all of the bases, but it was just not possible.

"I felt there was a stigma for having to get therapeutic help. Other than my boss, I certainly didn't share that with other people that I worked with. And I didn't feel I could even tell my sisters. Part of that was a feeling that I'm the oldest, the trailblazer who can forge through anything. The stigma of being in therapy implied that I'm weak. So, yeah, even while in therapy I felt that.

"But it got to a point where it was bad enough that the stigma was outweighed by the opportunity to get better. I didn't like the direction that things were going. Now maybe I would never have gotten to be totally agoraphobic, but I knew I didn't want to.

"I still have to carry the 'insurance' medication, so in the sense of being 'cured' all the way back to how I was before any of this happened—no. Therapy hasn't cured that. Some things have happened that have changed me forever, and all it can be is as good as it can be from now in the face of all of those experiences. Therapy has done wonders there for me.

"As for personal characteristics, I have an inquisitive mind. A thirst for knowing more about a situation or condition. I think wanting to know more about *me*. Eventually being able to open up and talk to somebody about things that I probably would have preferred to stay buried, but knowing that they couldn't if I were going to make progress. Maybe the ability to listen, not interrupt the therapist, but let them get their thoughts out. And for me, one of the traits was to take a lot of notes to refer back to. And questioning—there were times when a therapist would say something that I didn't quite understand, so not being reluctant to question the therapist was a quality that helped me."

Being Afraid to Open Up

Allen felt his inquisitive nature contributed to his good result in therapy. He said, "I think wanting to know more about me" helped to offset the stigma. Once past the fear, how interesting it is to learn about our minds and bodies—our *selves*. He spoke of "eventually being able to open up," because we don't tell all in the first visit. In fact, some of us might not tell all in the first ten or twenty years. Or ever.

In *The Noonday Demon,* Andrew Solomon tells about being at a weekend party where a woman, on learning that he was writing a book about depression, took him aside and confided that she was seeing a psychiatrist for depression. She asked him not to tell her husband. The next day, the husband, on learning the author was writing a book about depression, confided that he, too, was being treated for depression, but not to tell his wife because she wouldn't understand.[25]

Wouldn't it be good news if in therapy (because it hadn't happened in the marriage) each partner, in time, could learn to feel safe *within* themselves and then be able to share with each other their deepest feelings, including their shame? At first this seems just an ironic, maybe even humorous story. But it says so much about how hard it is to reveal our secrets, about the shame we feel at being weak or imperfect or different, about our deep need to hide the truth from others and to feel safe. What a poignant reminder of how difficult it is to talk—especially about what we don't want anyone else to know about us.

Allen said another quality that helped him in his therapy was "being able to open up and talk to somebody about things that I probably would have preferred to stay buried, but knowing that they couldn't if I were going to make progress." First there must be the awareness of things we don't wish to talk about and then an awareness of not feeling safe enough; self-awareness sometimes has to overcome a need to talk only about superficialities before we feel safe enough to talk about what matters. We must be patient with ourselves.

Talking: it sounds so simple.

NIMH Agoraphobia

Agoraphobia involves intense fear and anxiety of any place or situation where escape might be difficult, leading to avoidance of situations such as being alone outside of the home; traveling in a car, bus, or airplane; or being in a crowded area. About 0.8% of the U.S. adult population suffers with it; 40.6% of these cases are classified as severe. Of those with the disorder, 45.8% are receiving treatment, though for 41.2% of these it is deemed minimally adequate. Average age of onset is 20.[26]

Nora

Nora and her daughter saw the same therapist separately for a year. Nora believes they both benefited from learning better ways to communicate, a skill that transferred to other areas of their lives. She said that her curiosity and longing to understand their relationship better were incentives to examine their issues with a professional.

"I was actually curious—I've always been a curious person about people's thoughts and what makes people do things. I don't think people realize that their reactions to other people are related to earlier relationships, that something back there is causing you to be biased because of the environment you grew up in. The mind is very complicated.

"We all have backslides, but it's up to the recipient of the therapy, ultimately, to make the decision to change. It's so easy to blame someone else: 'Well, it was my mother's fault,' she laughs. "Maybe therapy worked for me because of my willingness to solve a problem and my deep desire to be closer to my daughter—and, I think, being able to admit there was a problem."

Admitting There's a Problem

Nora's comment of "being able to admit there was a problem" was so quiet it nearly slipped past unnoticed. The reason this can be so hard to do is that we retreat from whatever we don't want to know or remember. It could be to speak of an earlier loss or admit to a parent's meanness or indifference to us; these are painful conversations. We set up a barricade against knowing what is driving us to assorted unwelcome and self-defeating behaviors in the form of "little" obsessions, compulsions, addictions, sleeping problems, or eating disorders, to name a few, telling ourselves they're "not that bad."

Several memories may cluster behind the barricade. Instead of finding the courage to face what is there, we hide, concoct excuses, decide against therapy, or withdraw from others; anything to maintain the status quo and the façade that all is well. The barricade is stronger than nearly anything an army could devise, and we will do nearly anything to avoid knowing what is behind it, ignoring the pleas of those who love us and can plainly see our refusal to get acquainted with what is on the other side. Some keep the barricade in place throughout a lifetime. That's why a therapist's quiet, sustaining presence can make it possible to look within and be freed of the stranglehold such avoidance has on our life.

Nora is aware of "something back there" in relationships from an earlier time in her life as they influence the person she is today. While she acknowledges how complicated our minds are, those memories are not mentioned as being part of her therapy. Instead, the focus was on changes to her thinking, which resulted in an improved relationship with her daughter. What she learned has proven useful in many other areas of her life, but it all began with admitting there was a problem.

Melanie

Melanie waited twelve years to resume therapy after her first counselor accepted her sister as a client. Now with a therapist who understands her broad, multicultural interests, she feels relatively secure in a competitive profession. Her focus in therapy has shifted to relationships and self-esteem, though her comments here mostly concern her initial experience in therapy.

"My family was against my being in treatment. I didn't go home for the holidays for a number of years and instead made vacation plans. This was so I could develop autonomy. I had to express that I was not their puppet any longer and didn't even have to be a part of the family.

"I've talked about how bad my self-esteem is, but I think that one of the reasons I was able to seek help was because I had enough self-esteem. Still, I have this conflict within myself of needing help and not needing help. But I have to say, if I hadn't had that traumatic situation with a boyfriend, where I was having basically a mental breakdown, maybe I wouldn't have gone. It put me in a desperate situation and I was willing to try anything."

Caring Enough

Given her family's objections, it's not hard to see how difficult it was for Melanie to go into therapy. One comment that struck me was that even though she sought therapy because of poor self-esteem, it was having a sufficient amount of it that enabled her to go for help. Despite this insight, she continues to be in conflict about "needing help and not needing help." It seems that by choosing therapy she made a statement that she cared enough about herself to be saved from the confinement of being her parents' ever dutiful daughter.

She also mentions that for several years she didn't join her family for holidays and vacations. While deeply engrossed in the therapeutic process, we may distance ourselves from our families. If love is faithful, those who truly care about us will give us space and time without judgment or penalty; if they don't, that tells us something too.

Claire

Claire's mother was unable to be a nurturing support to her daughter. Initially, Claire believed that therapy would consist of intellectual discussions. She was quickly dissuaded from this notion. Therapy became a process of self-discovery as she sought to answer a question she had never been asked: "What do you want?" It was a beacon of light.

"I felt I needed therapy so badly that it wouldn't have bothered me if I had felt stigmatized. I didn't tell the whole world—I just told people I knew and trusted.

"The shame was more about the things I had done in my life. I felt ashamed, obviously, of having an illegitimate child, about some of the relationships that I got into with men, but I learned not to be ashamed because it was the result of everything that had happened to me as a child.

"I could give a parallel in the way that somebody who may be an alcoholic is ashamed of drinking. I was ashamed of other personal things in my life, because I knew I shouldn't be doing them, whereas to me a stigma is a mark that is placed on you externally by society. I've never been a person that cared a great deal about what society thought about me. That sounds the opposite of what I say sometimes about always trying to please people, but I think the always trying to please was about wanting approval and seeking the love and attention that I hadn't got as a child.

"Not feeling good emotionally until so late in life has stood in the way of my maybe developing my career, my other interests. I feel regret that if I hadn't grown up with this dysfunctional family and with the problems that I had, I could have made so much more of my life. I just wish that I'd got into therapy earlier.

"Other than the fact that I probably know more about myself than somebody who is mentally healthy and hasn't been through therapy, there have been no compensations for the circumstances of my life.

"Maybe some of the reasons therapy worked for me are that I'm tenacious and don't like to give up. That helped me stick with it. The fact that I was so bright got in the way of my therapy sometimes because I'd try to intellectualize it rather than get in touch with the feelings."

Relieving Soul Pain

Claire was fairly certain that the shame she felt was not about being in therapy but rather about things she had done, and that any stigma she might have felt was overcome by the urgency of her need to get help. And yet, she also recognized that she probably would not have made choices in her life that compounded, in some ways, her difficulties, if she had received the love and attention that she needed as a child. Though deeply grateful for the improvements therapy brought to her life, she was clear that they didn't compensate for what she lost.

In the midst of therapy, with the unexpected intensity of feelings bouncing off the walls, we don't notice everything that's going on. So this perspective from a distance reveals details and contours of the experience that we hadn't noticed passing through. Also, we may not have put into words before how we felt about something or how much it means to us.

Sometimes pain presses so persistently that it becomes like wallpaper in our minds, not as obvious or inescapable as a migraine, yet so ever-present it becomes part of our mental landscape. One example would be a feeling that you are always somehow less than others, someone less worthy, less gifted, less desirable. The feeling is so persistent that it becomes part of your idea of yourself. Then one day, after lots of work in therapy, you find you no longer feel that way about yourself; in fact, no longer *need* to feel that way about yourself. That's how it feels to relieve pain in one's soul.

It may be that an index of our well-being is in our answer to an impossible question: If you could live the live you have had over again, would you? It is possible, even likely, that talking to someone will bring enough relief of soul pain to want to live. This idea reminds me of the title of Robert Frost's poem, "Happiness Makes Up in Height for What It Lacks in Length."

NIMH Mental Illness Exacts Heavy Toll, Beginning in Youth

Researchers...have found that half of all lifetime cases of mental illness begin by age 14, and that despite effective treatments, there are long delays sometimes decades between first onset of symptoms and when people seek and receive treatment. The study also reveals that an untreated mental disorder can lead to a more severe, more difficult to treat illness, and to the development of co-occurring mental illnesses.[27]

Rose

Rose described her long struggle to get in touch with a small child's grief over her father's sudden death. Even now her emotions tend to be expressed more easily in physical ways other than being able to cry. She described the surprises—she calls them "insights" that come into the therapeutic setting—as the most important part of the work. Developing a sense of self stood out as a crucial milestone in her therapy.

"It was difficult to remain in treatment every time I called him [therapist] up and said I was quitting. . . . This is a very severe analogy, but I have been severely depressed and severely miserable, and I have thought many times I wish I weren't here anymore. But I never went so far as to think how I would do it. There may have been many, many times when I wanted to stop therapy, but I never did."

As she describes in retrospect her reasons for going into therapy, it's possible to see how therapy addressed contradictory ideas she had about herself, which later evolved into something more.

"I needed therapy because my life was falling apart, and I was doing things that I couldn't come to grips with in myself. My behavior was not matching the behavior of the person I thought I was, so I went into treatment because I was just not who I thought I should be or was or wanted to be. I was being treated badly by my husband. I didn't know what else to do. I couldn't rely on my parents for anything—they're the ones who got me there. My life was in shambles, and I was very young.

"I don't think I've ever felt stigmatized by being in treatment. I only talked about it with the people I thought it would be okay with, the people I felt that I needed their approval, but not from the outer world. My mother once called my therapist 'Mr. God' in a letter that she wrote to me, so I'm sure she had a lot of problems with it.

"Maybe in the early years I might have thought about the time and money I spent on therapy, but I never really have. It's just always been so necessary.

"When I first started therapy I spent a great deal of time at the bookstore looking for anything and everything that I could find myself in . . . Now I don't do that anymore. It's just not what I'm interested in doing. But I had to do that for a long time."

The stresses of Rose's childhood led her to years in therapy. I asked whether she felt compensated for the struggle to put her emotional life in order. She said, "The ability to deal with a very overbearing mother, make distinctions regarding friendships and my own needs, and working—supporting myself after never having been to college—teaching myself, so to speak, hearing myself talk, sorting it all out, finding my way to the other side: this has been a great compensation, a great gift one can give to oneself if one is willing to realize how valuable the difficult process can be."

Even though she has worked very hard to find her way from a life "in shambles," as she put it, "to the other side," she feels compensated by what she has learned.

Looking for Ourselves

Sometimes, during an in-depth therapy or analysis, we may develop for the first time in our lives a viable sense of self. Without one we are ill-prepared to meet life's demands, unable to hold up under the stresses placed upon us. Early and severe trauma, or an environment that is unstable, violent, or unpredictable, sets the stage for a lifetime of problems. Without a secure foundation—meaning free from danger or attack, free from loss or risk, from overwhelming fear, anxiety and doubt—we grow up to have a personality structure that is cracked and wobbly. Later trauma compounds the earlier ones, placing us ever more at risk in being able to keep ourselves together without a sufficient base of support.

Rose says, "I spent a great deal of time at the bookstore looking for anything and everything that I could find myself in…" We can feel within ourselves that something is missing. We look for pieces of ourselves outside of us, in books or in unhealthy attachments to others, rather than within us, as if there is no axis, only spinning round. There has been no long-term, dependable, stable, nurturing presence in these lives.

Rose commented that the early loss of her father and the absence of an opportunity to grieve left her with an incomplete sense of self: "What did I know? It was my mother's loss, not my loss. I was *only five*." As she grew up her life was filled with stormy family relationships, a troubled marriage, inadequate nurturing from an overbearing, competitive mother, and chronic health problems. Through it all has been the need to grieve.

It is profoundly consoling to have one's feelings believed and cared about, to be allowed to say them aloud, to weep, and to have someone understand, even feelings from long ago, deeply buried. Grieving lasts for as long as we are *not* allowed to have it.

A therapist does not impose ideas on us from folk wisdom, religion, or purveyors of advice about how we are to live. Our feelings are allowed to come forth in their raw, clear, and most human form. Given space and time, and a loving person who listens and feels along with us, grief runs its course. In this mighty relationship is the chance to experience at last our feelings so as to feel ourselves alive, even to want to live.

A therapist does not tell us what to do next in therapy or how we should feel. We learn to name our feelings, moor them to something within us, and discern subtleties between them. A good therapist would never say, as a directive, "Now it is time to grieve for the loss of your father," but waits for us to find the feelings in ourselves.

Each of us must locate the sources of our grief. No one can do it for us, and no one can tell us where they lie. The therapist verifies what we find, listening as we search for a lost mother, understanding what happened when we were young and one of our parents, or both, were lost to us, or some other calamity befell a child too young to withstand the blow. A therapist understands the ways these experiences limit us, limit our being able to be close to other people or to get around in the world.

Grieving for a cruel or careless parent is difficult—different from grieving for someone you loved and whose love for you was felt and cherished. It is a grief wrapped in guilt and anger. We may remain in therapy because it is the only place, physically and psychologically, to which we can dependably return to experience and tend to our feelings. The outside world has no patience with our needs. We can turn to literature, music, art, or religion to look for the feelings we need to reclaim, but in our therapist's office their readiness quickens. The release brings incomparable relief. In time we begin to make sense to ourselves, or sometimes even to have a self at all.

Rose found her *self*, letting it be nurtured and unfold in the warm light of a therapeutic relationship. Sometimes we don't realize what has happened to us, before therapy and during, until many years later.

Jenny

Jenny described the pain of abuse in her childhood, the death of her infant daughter, her struggles with depression and an eating disorder, and the frustrations of therapy. She is keenly aware of the stigma associated with having emotional problems. Despite the weight of her memories, she is undeterred in her quest to heal from the abuses of her past.

"I continue to feel that stigma of seeing a therapist from people, even friends. It's kind of that look in the back of their eyes, 'Oh, yeah, you're the sick one.' Or, 'Oh, yeah, you're the weak one.' Or, 'Why don't you just get over it?' Which seems to be a mantra of ignorant people." She laughs. "I refuse to bow to that stigma."

"They love me, but I still feel a stigma. People are uncomfortable with it. If I were to put a percentage on it, I'd say ninety-eight percent of people are uncomfortable with mental illness in general. They can hold it *out here*, because it doesn't touch *them*. It's not *their* problem.

"With sex abuse, they can't hold it *out here* because that's something that has or could affect everyone in one way or another. What I mean is, okay, say none of my group of friends has been abused or has a family member that's been abused, but they know me. And I bring that to the table whether I talk about it or not. Or they have a friend or their spouse has been abused and they don't know it yet...It's not something that you can hold *out here.* Whereas you can hold schizophrenia *out here.* Okay, a certain segment of the population gets this, it's a mental disease, it doesn't affect me. They can look at *that* comfortably. I don't think they can look at childhood sex abuse in that way. They can talk about rape and depersonalize that, but child sex abuse you can't. Because even if you're not touched by it, if you have a child, you think about it.

"I'm having a difficult time right now remaining in treatment. I had a difficult time at the beginning with this therapist because I didn't trust him or anyone. The difficulty was and continues to be the fear of facing myself and my stuff.

"I don't think anybody who experienced what I experienced could deal with it on their own. They might have managed to push it down, hide or mask it, or find another way to numb themselves. I do not believe there is one person in this world that could deal with the kind of things I experienced without getting therapy. And I don't mean just not be healthy without getting therapy; I mean not deal with life without getting therapy. In any real way. And what I mean by real way is to have real relationships. Do meaningful things. At least most of the time. Have children. Be a good parent.

"I'm trying to make myself whole again, and I've not done it. I think that one's psyche sets the pace. I'm going at it, at times, at a pretty clipped pace, but I have a lot of stuff to work through. I have thousands of traumas to work through. You know, some people get raped, and they have one trauma, and it takes them two years to work through it. Not to belittle that, but add getting raped four times a week—by your parents—that's a lot of trauma. I don't judge myself harshly for being in therapy for so long.

"I hurt on a regular basis at not having a family, not having a mom, not having anyone who really knows you and is there for you and loves you unconditionally, and you can get mad at and they still love you. I don't have that. I never had that. And I feel that big hole in my life, and I need to try to satisfy that somehow. But . . ."

Her voice trailed off, then she resumed.

"Therapy hasn't cured my eating disorder, but I believe therapy might help me with that. I guess I'm not ready to be cured from that yet. I need it, still. It kind of anaesthetizes you. It's another way of numbing yourself, when you don't eat. The hunger pains overwhelm the emotional pain, so I'd rather feel the hunger pain. I still need those tools right now. Not all the time, but I do. It's a defense. That's why some days I *have* to purge. Have to. Need to. And other days, I don't, I'm fine.

"I feel that with time my eating disorder will work out. One thing at a time. I've got a lot of really big things to work on, and granted that's a dangerous aspect to my life, and probably sooner the better that I deal with it, but I'm sure it will work out.

After a few moments, she added, "My stepfather left when I was 12. She married someone else right away. He [the third husband] was a real bastard. First thing he said to me when I met him was, 'I hate kids.' I'm 12. This guy is moving into my life. She married him three months after . . . and once, before they were married, she took me, dropped me off at my stepfather's so she could have the afternoon with her new boyfriend. So I got to be raped one more time."

"I've always known there was fondling, and I always felt as if I didn't belong anywhere, like I was a fake, and someone was going to find me out, but when I first started realizing, it unwrapped itself over a few years. But when I realized the implication of it in my life, how it affected my life, it took me awhile. After I realized what happened to me, it took me awhile to see the implication—and I'm still seeing it. It's a learning process. I'll probably come across things all my life. 'Oh, that's why I don't like yellow, because my mom loves yellow!' I hate yellow! It's my most unfavorite color. That makes sense!" she laughs.

"I bring stubbornness to my therapy. A sense of responsibility—more toward my son than toward myself. A need to be happy. I'm very tenacious. If I set my mind to something, that's what's going to happen."

When I asked people if they felt in any way compensated for the emotional problems of their lives, some of them seemed puzzled by my question. That was not the case for others, including Jenny.

"I have a sense of pride that I survived. I wouldn't say there's a balance, there certainly isn't. But I have this beautiful son who is truly a gift from God. He is so special. I feel like that's compensation. I feel like [her infant daughter] was compensation. Even though she died, she brought a lot to my life. She opened the door to my grief. . . . And I feel compensated when I am able to help someone. When I'm able to reach someone on a level that other people can't because I have felt what they're feeling. That's a gift, I feel."

Seeing through a Clearer Lens

In "afterthoughts" about therapy, Jenny could express herself so vividly because therapy had rendered her no longer mute. When she said the death of her infant daughter was a gift ("She opened the door to my grief.") it showed how events today can be emotionally powered by events in the past. In the course of her therapy, up until her baby's death, she had been unable to feel the grief she had stored somewhere in the depths of her being.

She also points to feelings she found as she wrestled with parts of herself she didn't want to face. She sees her eating disorder as a way of numbing herself, a way of acting out the pain she can't yet locate in herself nor yet put into words.

She also quietly comments about the slow unwrapping of her awareness of the extent to which she had been abused by her sister, mother, and stepfather. She says her psyche sets the pace at which she can allow herself to realize the effects of what happened.

Many of those who have a history of sexual abuse will enter therapy without even realizing that they were abused. Certainly we have no knowledge of the ways these experiences have shaped us. We might think of this as analogous to lead or asbestos poisoning, where injuries do not appear for many years (as opposed to an auto accident, where injury is quickly apparent). But children and young adults know nothing about the damage from childhood molestation and abuse in its many forms. As with other kinds of trauma, we dissociate ourselves from it for years. Even knowing what happened, we blame ourselves, only to find that decades later we are still dealing with its effects.

From such experiences our view of reality becomes distorted, yet we do not see the distortion. In therapy we begin to see—ourselves, our experiences—through a clearer lens. As long as we cleave to the myths we drape around our view, we will not see the painful truth nor emerge into its sunlight. Clear sight—and the enlarged emotional capacities that come with it—are compensation for some of us.

NIMH Long-Term Effects of Childhood Maltreatment

The long-term impacts of childhood maltreatment include higher rates of unemployment, poverty, and use of social services in adulthood...The related losses in productivity and tax revenues, increased spending on social services, and potential transmission of abusive behaviors from one generation to the next, suggest major costs to society as well.[28]

Beth

Beth felt she came to her first experience in therapy through a back door. In graduate school she had consulted a professor, who was also a therapist, with questions about her career. Gradually she realized she had come wanting therapy. She saw this person for a few years, then, after a hiatus of several years, she came by a more direct route to a new therapist. As a therapist herself, she deeply values the perspective she gains from being in "the other" chair. We learn more about her perspective on the therapeutic process in a subsequent chapter.

As Beth said, "I have learned about myself, more in my second therapy because it's clearer and more recent, and I'm finally starting to believe that I am not as messed up as I think I am. That I am not as bad a person that I think I am. That I have good qualities—I'm competent and capable. I'm a good person and smart—all these things. I'm starting to really recognize those things, which surprisingly is a difficult recognition for me to hang onto because it is unfamiliar and new. I think there is that tendency to want to cling to what is familiar even though it's a distorted, hurtful version of myself. Somehow that's what I know, and as I'm recognizing these more positive things, they're feeling uncomfortable. I'm not pushing them away, but I'm not embracing them. I'm fighting myself.

"It's probably difficult at times to stay in treatment when I've felt hurt. Pardon my language—should I just say, 'F— it. F— them.' You know? 'They hurt me, and I'm out of here.' Other than the times I feel hurt, I don't have any difficulty remaining in therapy, and I don't feel any stigma about seeing a therapist.

"Some people don't want to know about themselves. It's painful, it's embarrassing. Again, once you know something, you know it. People have various levels of wanting to understand themselves and their experiences, and how they've shaped them to be the person that they are, and to be comfortable. I don't know if that's quite the right word, but to be comfortable with wanting to go through that process. 'Who am I? How did I get to be this way?' We've got to look back in order to look forward, and we have various reactions to that. To me, that makes the difference between someone who will seek help and someone who won't.

"What I bring to therapy is this—I'm interested in knowing more about myself. Period. As difficult as that can be, and as exciting as that can be, and a whole host of experiences—I *want* to know more about myself. And I think that helps."

Revising Ideas about Ourselves

Beth said therapy has given her the chance to revise ideas she has about herself. She was aware of how, like a tight shoe, they impinged on her movement in life. She knew good things about herself, yet held on to the negative ideas, continually fighting these two poles. She knows that holding on to a "distorted, hurtful version of herself" keeps her from feeling more at peace and from other achievements and satisfactions as well. She also recognizes that not everyone is interested in getting to know themselves in the way that therapy makes possible.

I wondered how many people in the world live with a "distorted, hurtful version" of themselves, how many could be relieved of its burden and could live less encumbered with a "revised version." Because therapy largely belongs in the realm of a stigmatized choice (and one that too few people can afford), it is not widely recognized how much more alive one could feel after some concerted effort with a good therapist.

I read again how easily she says, "People have various levels of *wanting* to understand themselves and their experiences, and how they've shaped them to be the person that they are, and to be comfortable . . . with *wanting* to go through that process. 'Who am I? How did I get to be this way?'" Some people do not want to return, while others of us are required to before we can live more fully in the present—or to be able to live at all. As a therapist, Beth's attitude of open curiosity is a commitment to continue reaching into her mind until she finds what she is looking for in herself; she admits how difficult it can be to sit on the other side, how much work it is to revise ideas we have about ourselves.

Summing Up

This chapter considered therapy from a longer perspective, as afterthoughts about the experience rather than how it felt to be in the midst of it. One idea was that therapy educates us emotionally in a way that transcends the visible world and brings us into deeper layers of self-knowledge. Appointments with a therapist gently held us accountable for what we might have preferred to avoid. The fear of opening up to someone could be overcome by a wish to know ourselves better. And we saw that some people were plagued by an awareness of stigma, while others seemed immune.

Beyond natural catastrophes and war, traumatic events of all kinds happen in families. We protect ourselves from the emotional knowledge of what occurred, thereby ushering in symptoms that on the surface appear inexplicable; these were defenses against knowing and against feeling. Trauma and its aftereffects can be so severe as to obliterate the wish to live; therapy can change that, but not overnight.

Although some people were puzzled by the question of being "compensated" for their struggle with emotional problems, others had thought deeply about it. Because of therapy everyone saw themselves through a clearer lens, and some commented that in retrospect they realized how their vision had been obscured and distorted. Also, personal qualities that supported therapeutic efforts were similar to those that helped in other endeavors: showing up, diligence, persistence, curiosity, a willingness to be open minded, wanting to know more about ourselves, and a sense of responsibility to become healthier for the sake of our children. We also needed courage to face ourselves as we struggled to revise negative ideas about ourselves and the ways these informed our behavior.

Chapter V will try to understand ways that therapy impinges on and modifies, expands and deepens relationships with family and friends, at work, and with our therapist.

Chapter V

Relationships with Family, Friends, Work, and Therapist

Transformation takes place in the context of a relationship.

Jim Jones, former chaplain
Illinois Youth Center, St. Charles, IL

THOSE of us who enter therapy because of a lost or troubled relationship open ourselves to possibility: of discovery, of going into closed chambers of the heart, of seeing ourselves and others anew. In talking with a therapist, we have the chance to study the threads woven into the cloth of all our relationships.

It means we are willing to shoulder some of the responsibility for things being as they are and unwilling to live distant from others. By exploring our feelings about a troubled relationship, even one that feels vaguely not quite right, we might restore it or put nagging feelings to rest. It's hard to face the unknown and impossible to know how things will turn out. Therapy draws up from our depths, like a bucket in a well, a mingling of humility, courage, love—and clarity.

The people I spoke with described ways that therapy brought changes and improvements in relationships with family members, friends, and work. On the periphery of the conversations were questions of faith, of letting others know we are in treatment, and whether a therapist has struck any "wrong notes."

If relationships were easy, there wouldn't be so much conflict, so many unhappy or failed marriages, so much effort to keep up appearances. Each of us brings baggage from the past, most of which we don't notice. Those of us who grew up in families that couldn't work things out—where those in power called the shots, where hurt was never healed, where silence and distance filled the empty spaces—didn't learn how it feels to be able to iron out differences between people. We can learn how in therapy.

Often, a difficult relationship becomes an impetus for seeking therapy; if not that, it becomes part of the work. Relationships define us and make life meaningful. When relationships suffer, a therapist helps to sort it out, even improving the one we have with ourselves; without it we will struggle continually to stay afloat.

Therapy may change all of our relationships: relinquishing some old friends and developing new ones, distancing ourselves from some people, working out old issues with others (where that is possible), and deepening our love toward others. We may find the work we want to do and hold fast our faith or lose it. Through it all, our therapist is a reference point as we bring order to our lives.

Sarah

"I've made lots of changes while I was going through therapy. Because I was changing, relationships with some girlfriends were changing. One girlfriend in particular needed therapy. She was always telling me her problems, and I'd say, 'Why don't you get some help?' Finally she did, but it didn't last long. It just got to a point where it damaged our relationship, because I was moving on and she wasn't. I feel sorry for people who won't get help.

"I would let close friends know I was in therapy. Family, no. My friends were positive, because most of my friends were in therapy also. No one ever had a negative thing to say about it. From my parents, there would have been disapproval, and I don't really tell my parents anything about what I do. They don't know how to take me now because, I think, my dad knew he had a way of getting at me. They sense that I am a stronger person now.

"Even though my family relationships were unhealthy, back then they were my parents, and I listened to them and was in their life more. Whereas now we barely speak, and I'm fine with this. My dad will call me every couple of months. With my mom it's on and off. Sometimes I'll call them. I used to feel like I had to, like the daughter thing to do. We don't talk as much, and we don't have anything in common, because I've changed, not them.

"In the past, I was more open about therapy, about telling people, but now I'm less so. I'm struggling now because I lost all my long-time friends pretty much, so I am in the process of building new friends. Therapy really had that much of an impact on the friendships I had. They wanted to complain about the same old thing and not do anything about it. I didn't feel from them any sense of growing or eagerness to be a better person or to change their life. I felt like I became more of a sounding board for their complaints, like I was their counselor, and it was a bad feeling. I felt I was being used that way by a couple of friends. One girlfriend would say, 'Wow, that therapist is really good,' and I'd say, 'Well, why don't you go?' But it was easier just to call me.

"Now I am more selective in finding friends. I have fewer friends, but they're good friends. As far as relationships with men, I know now how to pick them, or what to look for. I would trust my instincts more in a relationship. I always had them, but I never listened to them. I had one part of myself telling me no, and another part that would end up saying, 'Oh, it's you—you're the problem.' I had those messages from my parents.

"My relationship with Hank is better because with therapy we talk about our problems more, or we know the bad points that need help, and before we get to those, we try to work them out."

Being in Transition in Relationships

At the time of our conversation, Sarah found herself in a series of transitions: from her second marriage to a deepening relationship with Hank, from a job that didn't challenge her to one that expanded her talents, from being racked with self-doubt and low self-esteem to someone who was starting to count on certain strengths in herself. She became a manager at her workplace, a position that afforded ample opportunity to observe others from a different vantage point: "I can see where they are is where I used to be, and I avoid that." She worked hard through her sorrows and didn't want to listen to friends who would not try to change their lot in life.

When asked about "wrong notes" with any of her therapists, she explained that three (out of four) counselors "during my time" would talk about their own lives. The third one was going through a divorce from an alcoholic husband just as Sarah was. She felt that "some of the advice she offered I didn't think was real good" and should not have been brought up during her appointment. She even felt at times that she was helping out the therapist with some of her problems.

Sarah was the first person I talked with who brought up the idea of the sacrosanct nature of the appointment period. We deserve—and are paying for—a time that is devoted to our concerns alone. When the therapist infringes on that by talking about themselves or bringing their problems into the session, we justifiably resent it. Perhaps one viable gauge of the caliber of a therapist is the extent to which the person needs to talk about his or her problems with a patient. It is one reason (among many) we want to find a therapist who has dealt with his or her own issues in their own therapy, and not in ours.

Sarah commented about a friend who followed her example, went into therapy, then soon exited. The reasons for people leaving treatment are probably well known among therapists. Among them are being scared, not being supported sufficiently by either the therapist or someone influential in the patient's life, an inability to meet the costs, being neither curious nor miserable *enough*, being unwilling to relinquish control or spend money on therapy, or having a disappointing experience with a therapist.

But for those who try and leave, I wonder if sometimes their expectations were unrealistic at the outset. When therapy takes longer and is harder work than we expected, some of us might be inclined to give up too soon. Yet sometimes, with such intense involvement and commitment, we wake up one day and realize we are not the same person. By seeing things differently, our world has changed. We may look for other qualities in friends than we used to, may even find that people we were close to have traits or requirements we hadn't noticed before. This can be unsettling—or feel like an accomplishment.

For Sarah therapy was a compass to use while everything else was changing. It eased several transitions in her life until things settled into place.

Hank

"I let some people know I am in therapy, but not everybody. They think it's good that I've taken the initiative to make life better. I'm reluctant to tell somebody that I feel is close-minded about stuff like that. It wouldn't benefit me to tell somebody who was like that because they'd say, 'You're just crazy!' and blow it off. But somebody that can understand what I would tell them—I think I can tell which people would . . . like, I could say, *this* guy would never go to a counselor, I just know it. So I wouldn't even mention that I was going, because it would probably be a negative thing for me.

"How therapy has affected my relationships has all been positive, I guess because you're more aware of people's feelings. If I had never gone to therapy I would probably be more judgmental toward people.

"I can't say that there's been any relationship that's really turned around in any way. With Sarah and I, it takes a lot of work, continual work, but I can't say that any has turned around. It just makes all relationships a little better."

Looking Beneath the Surface

Without the help of a good therapist, we tend to have little awareness or understanding of the world that exists beneath the surface, a world beyond what we see and know. If you were to mention that you are bothered by something that happened in the family of your childhood, some might say, "But that happened a long time ago!" Those who understand little about their own emotional life are unlikely to understand anyone else's. They live with a kind of emotional disability and may never understand that even though something happened "a long time ago," it may hold the key to understanding a great deal.

Like old photographs, memories and feelings about what happened long ago have all been preserved. Talking about them in the light of our adult understanding and with a knowing interpreter enriches our inner world and all our relationships.

Christine

"All my close friends know that I've been in therapy and have bulimia. At first I felt uncomfortable saying it, but I don't anymore. It feels very natural. I'm not perfect, and I have to admit it, and they don't mind," she laughs. "My boyfriend was in counseling, too, I found out, which made me feel a lot better after telling him.

"The reason I told him was . . . I was with my boyfriend and my friend and her boyfriend. The guys are roommates. We were at their house, and we were watching this show, a really stupid show, and at one point they were making fun of bulimics. My boyfriend didn't know I had bulimia at the time, and I had gotten upset. I wanted to get up and leave, but I was afraid of making a scene.

"Later that day I said, 'I didn't think that was very funny,' and he said, 'Yeah, I know, it's a pretty obnoxious show.' And then I said, 'You know, it really offended me because I have bulimia.' Then he felt really bad, and he said, 'I'm so sorry.' Then he said, 'I've had problems, too, I've been to a counselor myself.' Then I felt a lot better after telling him. So it sort of became a bonding experience!" she laughs again.

"It took my boyfriend so long to tell me why he went into therapy in the first place. It took him five months, I think. Guys just don't like to talk!"

Telling Someone Brings Relief

After learning her boyfriend had seen a counselor, it took five months before he told her why. The male aversion to being in therapy or appearing "weak" (even to themselves, even if no one knows about it) permeates societies and, perhaps even more so, a military culture. In statistics available from the Veterans Administration, the number of military personnel from recent wars who committed suicide has steadily increased, exceeding the number who were killed in combat. As more soldiers succumb to post-traumatic stress disorder, efforts are under way to train more therapists to address the need.

In recent years, in some doctor's waiting room, I happened to read an interview about a man in a war-torn country who had suffered massive violence in terms of threats to his life, threats to the lives of his family, being witness to horrific violence, and ordered to commit atrocities himself. Eventually he escaped and found refuge in another country. As I recall, he underwent five years of treatment for nightmares and made two serious attempts at suicide.

Five years may sound like a long time to a young person who doesn't want to be in treatment, who wants to get on with life, but the grim reality is that five years is not a great deal of time to regroup after terrorizing experiences. One of the huge challenges is learning again how to trust; without it our relationships remain superficial, at best. We must hang in there with a therapist as the battle ensues to regain trust. By slow and steady steps we have to prove to ourselves again and again that our therapist can be trusted. This new information doesn't simply override what has been seared into memory.

Returning soldiers' relationships with family, friends and themselves can begin to recover when they bring themselves to talk with a therapist about what happened. Each conversation, each meeting with each memory, over time lessens the intensity of PTSD symptoms. Even with therapy, even with a lot of it, the memories, the anger, and the terror don't disappear. But they become less intense and more manageable, making it possible to live without being enslaved to a distorted sense of reality.

We read and hear about people who don't talk about what happened, who claim they just "move on." The question is whether these accounts of those who emerge unfazed offer a complete picture of the person's relationships and emotional life. It is hard to imagine moving on without sacrificing *something*, albeit something that may be invisible to others—or apparent to others, but not to oneself. The irony is that none of us can imagine how much better our lives will be until we go through the hell of remembrance to reach the other side of safety, trust, and normalcy. Without treatment, we are at risk of depending on destructive ways to keep our feelings in check, of becoming emotionally numb, cut off from many of life's joys in the service of hypervigilance.

NIMH Soldiers and Suicide

Today more soldiers are dying from suicide than combat. Suicides have traditionally been lower in the Army than in age and gender matched civilians. In 2004 the suicide rate in the U.S. Army began to climb, surpassing the civilian rate in 2008, and when combined with deaths from high-risk behavior, surpassing the mortality from combat in 2009. The suicide rate has continued to increase, with 164 deaths among active duty soldiers in 2011.[29]

Greg

"I don't remember if I told anyone I was in therapy. It wouldn't normally come up. I don't know that I would have purposely hidden it, but I don't recall if I mentioned it to anyone, or to my daughters. They were grown by then and out of the house.

"It's hard to have a good relationship with anybody if you're depressed. I couldn't have been much fun to live with if I'm depressed, so I'm sure it affects your relationship with your spouse. My wife happens to be sensitive to how people are doing and feeling, so I'm sure it was very noticeable to her, and she encouraged me to get therapy."

Finding the Truth of Our Feelings

Depression is stealthy; it steals the lilt from life. Because of its many disguises, we may not recognize it, not even in ourselves. If anyone suggests we're depressed, we deny it, unaware that we have become numb to our own feelings, living our lives on automatic pilot, and staying a safe distance from others.

Characteristics of depression are often listed on websites or in pamphlets on display at the drugstore. Less commonly known are its guises, ways we adapt our behavior to conceal (from others and ourselves) the fact that we are depressed. In these guises we might convert our depression into a physical symptom, such as an eating disorder, panic attack, or obsessive-compulsive tendencies; or excessive busyness, excessive talking, or anything to mask what is going on inside us and keep our focus trained outside ourselves. Depression interferes with relationships, whether we are aware of it or not.

In "Doonesbury," cartoonist Garry Trudeau delivered a series of comic takes on the plight of the returned soldier whose family, "battle buds," and doctor urge him to see a counselor. At their first meeting, the soldier tells the counselor that his wife threatened to "split" if he doesn't get help, and "my kid was afraid of me," but he insists he's fine.[30]

Such is the nature of numbness and denial for any of us and the plague of stigma—the fear of facing painful memories. With it comes an inability to be true to oneself nor fully honest with anyone else. Virtually all our effort goes into maintaining a pretense that all is well.

Allen

"The only people who knew I was in therapy were my wife Sharon and my boss, who needed to know because sessions had to be scheduled during working hours. My employer was quite understanding and actually encouraging. I was lucky.

"I mostly tried not to mention it. To this day, I don't think I've ever told anybody. I mentioned to my sisters that I am subject to anxiety attacks. I found it comfortable to do so as I learned more about myself and became more accepting of who I am. And they didn't react negatively at all. But in terms of actually telling folks that I've been in therapy, I just haven't. But with Sharon, it was important to me that our relationship be based on honesty. I wanted her to know what she was getting into. If it was going to make a difference, that wasn't something that should be kept a secret.

"Because of therapy I've been able to share a life with Sharon that isn't cloistered. It helped me address things about my panic attacks. Our times together have been enriched because I don't have to say no to invitations. We've had super times with our kids and their families. And that's been influenced by the therapy. Without it, I'd still be shying away from social situations."

Preserving Privacy and Personal Dignity

Allen, like many of us, had been secretive about his emotional problems and therapy—going around in fear that someone might find out, being on the alert, being careful that no one knows. But his wife knew, and being honest with her was what mattered.

Each person must decide how much to disclose to others about what is essentially a private matter. We have to figure out what is to be gained by telling and what is lost by being secretive, and the effect on our relationships of disclosure or concealment. It depends on the culture around each individual's life, but as we become more comfortable with ourselves and with the knowledge of having faced down the enemy within, telling becomes a little easier, at least in certain settings. It's possible that intense privacy in this matter also belies a reluctance to trust, as if making yourself vulnerable could be used against you. Each person's sense of what constitutes personal dignity is worthy of respect.

NIMH Social Phobias

Social phobia is a strong fear of being judged by others and of being embarrassed. This fear can be so strong that it gets in the way of going to work or school or doing other everyday things...Most people who have social phobia know that they shouldn't be as afraid as they are, but they can't control their fear. Sometimes, they end up staying away from places or events where they think they might have to do something that will embarrass them.[31]

James

"Even though I wasn't dealing with issues like sexuality and self-acceptance, having already come out, I still was trying to live honestly, trying to do the right thing. Therapy definitely improved relationships with my family because I became more patient with them. I became more forgiving and allowed people to handle things and respond in their own way, knowing that that's them, as opposed to being frustrated with not liking the way people respond. I learned I wasn't responsible for how someone else feels, but only for how I live my life and how it might affect others."

I asked James whether therapy had affected his life's work.

"I hadn't really thought of this before, but when I was in therapy, I didn't have my present business. I was still working in a family business that was very successful, but had run its course. I was faced with 'What am I going to do now with my life? What do I want to do?' My dream for a long time had been to have my own business, and it just so happened at that time that that door opened for me. I was still at the later stages of resolving my relationship with Daniel. His accident happened just before my thirtieth birthday. I was becoming independent from my relationship, independent from the family business, and growing into a new direction to a dream that I wanted. I never made the connection to therapy before, but it felt like a healthy flow and a start to something new."

Working Things Out to Become Free

Instead of walking out on his partner, therapy gave James the chance to resolve the relationship with Daniel and begin to come to terms with what had happened in their lives.

With it came quiet changes in self-awareness and in relation to his family. By becoming more independent, he was free to pursue a dream of having his own business. It's hard to see in ourselves that *this* part of us is connected to *that* part of us, like a web in which one part can't be eliminated or clamped without altering the whole. James' story illustrates this truth.

Of course it's possible that even without therapy James would have found his way into becoming a successful entrepreneur. Yet he felt it was not mere coincidence, that therapy had cleared reception of the work channel, helping him make sound decisions that led to greater satisfaction in his work and personal life. He is unlikely to become someone who ruefully says in his fifties that he doesn't know what he wants to be when he grows up.

Melanie

"My family had such a stigma about therapy. Basically I was the family scapegoat. I was deemed to have all this talent and beauty and grace—that anything anybody in the family wanted, they were pretty much free to take. If they borrowed my clothes, I was supposed to just say okay. I would be selfish if I didn't share them. When I had friends and introduced them to my sister, she automatically assumed that they were her friends, and she would ask them for things that were inappropriate to ask of your sister's friends—you would only ask that of your own friends. She had a hard time with that. It happened again when she began to see the same therapist. She didn't understand that this was *my* therapist.

"She told me she wouldn't go to therapy if I didn't allow her to go to my therapist, saying she wouldn't trust anyone else. We didn't have problems right away, but we did after a couple of years. My sister got a lot of benefit from it, but it started being a not-so-good thing for me. When I would bring this up to my therapist, she got really freaky that I was going to leave her. I know she felt a huge amount of guilt about it afterwards.

"I have a better relationship with my siblings now than I had before therapy. I'm very close to the sister that I shared a therapist with—now. She and I have something in common in that we both were in therapy. But even with my other siblings, I am less reactive and more able to set boundaries, which they respect. I probably have a better relationship with my parents, but that's because I don't talk to them about anything personal. From a certain point of view, you could say that I have *not* as good a relationship with them, but that's because when I set the boundaries, they refuse to follow them.

"It has made me respect myself better, and so people respect me better. Before therapy, I needed people to fit into clear categories of who they were. Now I let people set their own space. I have levels of friendships where I am very close to some and not so close to others, which allows for a wider group of friends.

"One of the things I'm seeking is to have close relationships with people where it's not that neurotic relationship that I created with my mother—which is a strong female person who ends up controlling you. Through the years, I've had a number of female friends that have very strong personalities, who want you to do what they say. At some point it falls apart, because it was a re-creation of my relationship with my mother. The quality of my relationships has changed. In some ways relationships have gotten less close, but in other ways they've gotten more full-spectrum; there's more going on with relationships.

"I find meditation is helpful. It's a good start to therapy, because it's easier to take a look at what your thoughts are when your mind slows down. I consider them to be hand-in-hand. Before I was in therapy, when I would close my eyes, I would just get this barrage of pictures that would run through my head. It was very hard to have any sense of calm about me. When I started meditating, that started to calm down, so that's been a real help for me. Certainly my faith has been affected by my therapy—everything is affected by my therapy."

Understanding the Mechanics of Relationships

The stigma Melanie felt about being in therapy came from her family. She went anyway, and the picture she draws deepens the meaning of personal boundaries. Her siblings were accustomed to being allowed to take whatever they wished and nothing really belonged only to her. Out in the world as an adult, it's easy to imagine feeling at sea, unprotected, not being clear whether or not anything could belong to her, wondering if she's being selfish, and feeling vaguely guilty about it—yet all the while being unaware of forces in the family which have shaped her feelings and ideas. When she begins to talk and remember, the picture of what it was like begins to emerge.

Small wonder that it's a lot of work in therapy to become *aware* of the ways these circumstances shape us, then to learn how to set limits on others, and to begin to allow yourself to feel you have certain rights as an individual. I could feel how hard it was for Melanie to say no to her sister, and what an achievement it was to recognize the feeling of being violated (in a certain way), then to learn to stand up for herself—and how this must have contributed to her self-esteem.

Melanie's story also shows how the dynamic that is set up in a family spills into one's life as an adult in trying to navigate the unspoken rules of friendship when vision is fuzzy. This sense *of how things are done* is woven into the fabric of one's self in those first lessons that small children are so intent to learn. Through her story we can imagine how hard it would be to figure out (on our own) why aspects of our relationships might tend to be derailed. And this miniature scene describes only one of countless variations that could explain why our relationships aren't going well.

When relationships repeatedly go awry, therapy helps us understand the mechanics of what we do or say, expectations we have, and ways of responding to others that may keep us from the pleasures of other people's affection and regard for us. What some people appear to do effortlessly, others of us have to labor at tirelessly, deconstructing scenarios from our memory bank then putting the pieces back together to try again.

Claire

"My mother did a lot of damage to me, and I repeatedly sought out similar personalities in personal and professional relationships. But I have used counseling to work on those issues to the point that I can laugh at my boss when he acts like my mother. My therapist encouraged me to react outwardly in the opposite way to what I was feeling. It was very hard to do, but the more I practice, the better I get at it. I find even those dysfunctional people treat me better as I change my behavior.

"There was never a 'wrong note' with my therapist. He was a very special man. I mean, it's part of the therapy process that you get angry with your therapist sometimes, and I did, which helped me get in touch with my anger. But there was never anything that was 'off the mark.'

"Had I grown up with a normal family and without all the problems I grew up with, I think that, given my intellect and abilities, I could have been more in touch with what I wanted to do and had the time and energy to pursue those things. So I think that my life's work has been very affected by my mental health issues, because the things that I did were very much beneath my abilities. I just didn't have the emotional ability to pursue either the education or the confidence in myself to do them, and so my life's work could have been very different had circumstances been different.

"In terms of relationships with family, some are better, some are worse, some are nonexistent now, by my choosing—with my mother, certainly, because she was the cause of most of my problems. For years I struggled with feeling I ought to have a relationship with her because she was my mother, because she gave birth to me despite her problems. Finally I decided that it wasn't going to work. I just don't have anything to do with her now, and it's a relief.

"My relationship with my father has gotten better mainly because he had to find a way to stay in touch with me without her knowledge. So we have gotten to know and understand one another better. We've been able to develop a relationship, which we never had much of before.

"My brother and I were close for a long time, and toward the end of therapy, he went through some of his own problems, and we had a major fight. We did get over it, but we don't have the same close relationship as before. Part of me thinks that I was his little mother in a way, growing up. I felt I had to take on all his problems, too. Now that I'm not so willing to take on all of his problems—I think sometimes you change and other people don't—because you're not interacting with them in the way that you've interacted all your life, that is hard for them. I don't think that we have . . . I almost hesitate to use the expression 'as good a relationship as before,' rather, I don't *feel* as good about our relationship as I did before. But that's okay, because I understand why.

"I've weeded out friends that I decided were negative relationships in my life. With others, there were difficult times, especially when I was going through a difficult time in therapy. For the most part, we have weathered them and got through them, and our friendships are stronger. But those are mainly people that I find are more the kind of people that I would have sought out after therapy. Now I tend to seek out better relationships. And my therapist told me that would happen.

"I know that after therapy I would go home and my family would try to relate to me the way they always had. It didn't work because I had changed so much. My mother always went out of her way to make my visit unpleasant and on my last trip I finally realized, because I didn't see her, that she couldn't stand it that I was the center of attention when I went home because she always had to be the center of attention. I mentioned it to my father and he said, 'Oh, yes!'"

I asked Claire if she recalled a time where her employment had been affected by her therapy.

"Once when I was in a job where I had been the meek, eager-to-please little girl that I was before I went into therapy—because of the stage I was at in my therapy, I was just learning to express my anger—I did not express my anger in the best way. When it happens today I can deal with it more professionally. It led to my termination in that job, but I can't say that was a wholly bad thing," she laughs.

Getting Beyond Loneliness

Growing up in a family that fails to nurture and protect the children leaves them physically and emotionally compromised. Some fortunate children tend to be more "stress resistant." With others, the family cobbles together sufficient support for each of its members. But those who grow up under great stress and without enough support may end up walking a lonely road throughout their lives.

Support is a catch-all term. Under its umbrella are feelings of being safe, seeing ourselves reflected in a parent's loving eyes, being held and treated (mostly) with patience, being comforted and encouraged to become strong and independent, and being allowed to say how we feel.

Lives may be lonely for a lot of reasons. Being unable to trust others and needing to stay at a self-protective distance is one. We may keep trying to work out something from an earlier time in every subsequent relationship, till we give up on relationships altogether. Another is when a continuing attachment to one or both parents prevents other relationships from blossoming into maturity. We don't see ourselves objectively, nor the scaffolding that supports the ideas we have about ourselves, but those whose childhood development is supported from one stage to the next have a better chance of achieving substantial and satisfying relationships with others and in their life's work.

A parent's primary responsibilities are to nurture and protect a child. The stresses of life that are placed upon parents who are unable to fulfill their responsibilities adequately may put their children at risk. Claire points out some of the ways her life was affected by earlier relationships, especially with her mother, and these included low self-esteem, the educational level she achieved, depression and limited energy, health problems, difficult relationships past and present, being without direction or satisfying work, and self-defeating decisions. Despite it all, therapy and a measure of self-discipline helped her achieve a lifestyle that brought her both independence and satisfaction.

Close work with a good therapist helps people close developmental gaps so they can come closer to securing what they want in their lives, more free of the burdens of poor emotional and physical health.

NIMH Anxiety Disorders

Anxiety Disorders [panic, obsessive-compulsive, PTSD, social anxiety, phobias, and generalized anxiety disorders] affect about 40 million American adults age 18 years and older (about 18%) in a given year, causing them to be filled with fearfulness and uncertainty. Unlike the relatively mild, brief anxiety caused by a stressful event (such as speaking in public or a first date), anxiety disorders last at least 6 months and can get worse if they are not treated. Anxiety disorders commonly occur along with other mental or physical illnesses, including alcohol or substance abuse, which may mask anxiety symptoms or make them worse.[32]

Rose

"I let others know I'm in therapy, but I'm usually pretty careful about who I tell, so they're going to respond positively. It's not something that I talk about very much anymore. At one time I did, and maybe then I wanted to find out, 'Oh, God, how are they going to feel about this, and how are they going to feel about me,' but I don't worry about that anymore.

"I think it was hard on my kids when I was in therapy. On the other hand it was good for them, because I was able to use my therapist as a sort of ghost father so that when something would go wrong, I had somebody I could lean on and say, 'This is going on here. What am I going to do?' My mother and father didn't like it particularly that I was in therapy.

"In relationships, I'm more impatient in some ways than I might have been before. Sometimes I blame that on work, because I am spending so much time listening to other people about their work and their businesses, taking someone to lunch, and it can go on and on, and they're really only interested in talking about themselves, and there's no back-and-forth. I'm not willing to tolerate that in a relationship anymore. If it gets to be too one-sided, I'm not going to see that person so much.

"When my father died, my mother became the pet of the family. It was really always about her then. That need to take care of her was pervasive in my life. 'If only I could give her what she needed, then all would be well.' Consequently I grew up rather passive, and I think that without my therapist, I probably would still be that way, not wanting to ask anyone to pass the salt.

My mother could be fun, entertaining. And as long as I was compliant, we were great pals. It wasn't until I was married and had serious physical problems of my own, marital problems I couldn't face, that I began to realize how I had been her lackey.

"Over time I began to gravitate toward people that I felt could teach me something—things that my mother never did—about just living, risking, taking chances."

Filling a Parent's Needs

The job of parents is to fill their children's needs; the job of children is to be children who are allowed to grow up and become independent. But in some families children are asked to fill their parents' needs, sometimes for the rest of their lives.

Some parents, who were not themselves supported as children into maturity and strength, rely on their children (and adult children) to make up for what they missed. When we are children we are oblivious to the ways we fill our parents' needs, but as adults may chafe under a parent's continuing tight controls and short leashes.

Examples abound. A parent is always mysteriously ill to keep an adult child tending to rather endless needs. A father sees to it that his adult daughter accompanies him on trips and even errands, leaving her little chance to develop attachments with people her age. A mother keeps her son in touch with her daily by cell phone and little crises that require his help; she doesn't see that she has done anything wrong when he repeatedly loses his temper with her. A parent keeps an adult child attached to her by frequent (and irresistible) gifts of money and clothes, effectively blocking the adult child's sense of independence. Some parents use guilt to keep their kids connected to them.

Therapy heightens our awareness of facets of relationships we may have glossed over. A pair of more objective eyes views our situation from across the room, helping us find ways to undo some of the ties that bind. Working ourselves free of a parent's persistent hold requires dedication from therapist and patient, but such newly found freedom is worth the fight.

Jenny

Jenny's excerpt for this chapter is in two parts. She saw therapy as a way to make herself "whole again" after the traumatic events of her childhood, the realization of which "unwrapped itself," as she put it, over the course of years in treatment.

"I've been able to forgive some people on the periphery of all of this. I've been able to forgive my sister who was so angry as we were growing up. She victimized me a lot. She tried to kill me a couple of times, and would smother me with pillows. She used to have this rage that was frightening—unbelievably frightening. She would beat the hell out of me. I don't mean like little kids fighting, I mean like slamming my head on the floor repeatedly. I've been able to forgive her for that because I understand that she was being victimized, too, and she was just so angry, and I was the only person she had to take it out on. I had no one to take it out on, so I took it out on myself."

"I've been able to forgive my dad. I don't think without therapy that I would have been able to understand that he's this little boy in a grown up's body who has been terribly hurt himself, and he fears rejection more than anything. But the biggest reason that I've been able to forgive him is that he has said, 'I was a lousy dad, and I'm so sorry.' And I said, 'You know what, Daddy, yeah, you were. You were lousy. But let's go from here.' I always felt for the longest time—see, my mom's still alive—that if she would just own it, truly own it, take responsibility for it and apologize, that I could maybe have the mommy that I always wanted. But the reality is I'll never have it—I've never had it, I'll never have it. So, I've been able to forgive. I think that's a big one. If I could only forgive myself! I'm still working on that."

Our conversation shifted somewhat to the here-and-now as Jenny commented that the next day would be Mother's Day. She has no contact with her mother. Though her son asks about her occasionally, it is not as his grandmother. Jenny has told him that her mother is very sick, that it causes her to do mean things to people, that they are not punishing her mother by not being in contact, but are trying to protect themselves. She adds, "It took me awhile to work that one out. When he gets old enough, probably well into his teens, I'll tell him the truth. He probably will have guessed it by then."

Healing Relationships

No matter how old we are it is deeply human to want to feel love and admiration for our parents and to feel their love shining on us, even after they are gone. When something obstructs those feelings—something harmful they did, yet never acknowledged—we want to move it out of the path. We want to believe that forgiving them will bring them nearer to us and bring us peace.

There are people who readily forgive those who have hurt them, even grievously, without expecting contrition or apology. Others feel that, without having to take responsibility for what they did, we would be giving the offender tacit permission to hurt us with impunity, thereby relinquishing our human rights. Before someone can apologize or take responsibility, he has to be aware of having injured another person. We don't feel sorry for what we've done without first becoming aware of having caused someone pain, then aware of feelings of guilt; from such awareness contrition and humility may rise.

Jenny could forgive her father when he admitted he was not a good father. The story was different for her mother: "If she would just own it, and truly own it, take responsibility for it, and apologize." Apparently, like many people, her mother couldn't.

Some things are grievous enough that it is not for us to forgive. The effects of whatever happened to someone cannot be measured by the number of slaps, beatings, rapes, or insults. And even if they could, there are also the offenses that are less visible, that are done to the heart of a person, to their idea of themselves, and to their soul. These are things that are said and done to children that can make it nearly impossible for them to live. They have been branded by trauma as ranchers do with cattle. So although we may come to believe that we have nothing much to complain about (or people in our lives lead us to believe that), and we become convinced that things were "not that bad," these quiet events may be severely disabling psychologically.

Many injuries aren't reported to authorities because, for many years, they don't show. We are unaware of the connection between *that* and *this*. We only become aware when we can't get ourselves out of bed, can't stop drinking, lose our temper over "nothing," find we no longer want to live, or, having children of our own, suddenly one day understand something about *ourselves*. Then we begin to learn painful truths we would far rather not know.

It takes a great deal of courage to withstand the pain of recognizing some of the experiences and beloved figures that harmed us. It also takes a strong therapeutic relationship with someone who will help us explore our feelings. If we offer forgiveness, it should be authentically ours and not what someone else dictates.

NIMH Child and Adolescent Depression

Juvenile depression rarely exists in isolation, and children and adolescents with depression exhibit great variability in clinical characteristics (e.g., age of onset, course, severity), patterns of neurobiological correlates, and social profiles of risk. In addition, treatment response varies considerably among depressed youth.[33]

Jenny, continued

Jenny remembered a time when a therapist had struck a "wrong note," something that felt somehow not right. This referred both to an ethical issue and to a sense that the therapist was just not "getting it," was not understanding. Her experience is an example of a therapy that tried to override her natural defenses, which are in place after all to protect her, rather than letting memories return when she is ready to face them.

"There was one therapist who was working with my therapist briefly. The other therapist does this holographic imaging. It's another form of contacting your difficult memories and dispelling them from your body. And he had a seminar for a handful of women who are clients of my therapist, who was supposed to be a part of it and be there to offer support to us while this other therapist did his thing. We were all in a group, and that was the most awful, awful therapeutic experience I have ever had in my life. And I'm still angry about it.

"This other therapist had treated me a few times before with this holographic imaging, and it was fine. It wasn't as good as the EMDR, but I got some relief from it. What made me gravitate towards this guy was that it was almost like he could read me—what happened to me—just by looking at me. The first time he treated me, he told me several things that had happened to me as I was growing up, and it just wigged me out. 'He knows. He knows!' And I believe he did. But this man was more ego than therapist, and in the session, it was more about him giving his shtick, and he would bring us through these exercises. I don't know if you've ever been in a group setting like that, but it's really a bad idea. Because what happens is you've got all these—and I don't know that everybody was a sex abuse survivor—but everyone had their trauma, it was all trauma survivors—and so someone might talk about her issue, and that would trigger me off the wall—I'm having flashbacks all over the place—and nobody to tend to me. And so he kind of opened up all of our wounds, and . . . I mean, it was awful. I was having such a difficult time."

In the midst of this experience, the original therapist for all of these participants entered the hospital for emergency surgery and was unable to practice for two months while he recovered.

"So here I am with my guts hanging out, and my one stabilizing force nowhere. Unavailable. It was terrible. Terrible. And I was furious with him [the first therapist] because he kind of pushed me into it. And I was . . . I don't know, I don't know. I was furious with him about that.

"One aspect of the relationship with him is that money is a really big issue. He charges me for times he shouldn't. And I believe—and I'm sure I'm right—he was making money off of this. He was getting a cut. So I feel like he insisted that I go because he wanted the money. And that's actually why I haven't been to him in the last several weeks because I'm feeling . . . He did! I know he did! And it really bothers me. And actually that's one thing I need to talk to him about. I'm feeling used. And that made me feel very used, that he would . . . it's probably not fair to him, but I feel like he endangered my mental health for his own gain. And, you know, this guy hasn't been back. Everybody hated it. Everybody felt it was horrible. All of his clients who were there.

"I totally shut down after that. He wasn't available, so I just pulled right back inside of myself. It took months to get me back to where I had been.

"The money has been the one thing that has struck a wrong note. I feel very used a lot of times. I feel like I have to watch the bills, that he'll charge me if I don't watch everything, he'll charge me for stuff that he shouldn't. It's kind of the elephant in the room that I need to talk to him about. Because I've never out and out said it, and I need to say it."

While she was on the subject, Jenny drew forth another example of a wrong note with her therapist.

"Our marriage counselor now is another therapist. We had seen a different one for about seven months, and it was a complete waste. We quit. I said to my therapist, 'Do you have someone else?' He said, 'Yes, [our present marriage counselor]. Actually, this is who I thought of first when you asked me for a recommendation.' And I said, 'Then why didn't you give me her name?' Well, the one he first recommended us to was in his office, so he gets money from it. [Our present marriage counselor] is not in his office."

It felt, as if having been given the chance to talk freely about her feelings on the matter, Jenny put together a realization of issues that had been simmering for some time—all in response to my question of whether or not there had ever been a "wrong note" in the course of treatment.

"I need to talk to him about this because I'm pissed about it. So he sent us to this woman who he didn't necessarily think would be a nice match because it benefited him."

Vetting a Therapist

To "vet" a person is to evaluate someone thoroughly before placing trust in them. Each of us has to do that with any therapist we see, and as well anyone with whom we have a relationship. Some of us will have a more difficult time with this than others. In *Psychoanalytic Psychotherapy*, Nancy McWilliams writes, "Because the transferences of clients with histories of traumatic abuse tend initially to be intense and relatively undiluted by observing capacities, it is hard for such individuals to take in the possibility that a therapist sincerely has their best interests at heart. Trauma survivors mix us up more dramatically with the people who have hurt them than most patients do. The *slow process of differentiating the present from the past has always been the heart of the therapy experience* for such clients."[34] [italics mine] And so, for many of us, the process of vetting a therapist necessarily is repeated again and again. I would guess that a lot of people ditch therapy at these junctures rather than stick it out.

The holographic imaging therapy which Jenny described as "another form of contacting your difficult memories" felt like a form of emotional violence against her and the other participants. She was "wigged out" by the feeling that he could read her face and know what had happened to her, but it's possible that her own therapist had briefed the imaging therapist about all of his clients before the sessions began. In any case, it was hardly surprising that she shut down for months after the experience, nor that she feels she was being "used."

I find this story a frightening cautionary tale. Those who are drowning will grasp at anything to save themselves, and similarly, those who live with the emotional residue of severe trauma will grasp at nearly anything for relief from pain. But it takes time, for some of us decades, to learn to trust our therapist, patiently showing up and working through our memories inch by inch, layer by layer. I'm not sure a process as delicate as this can be by-passed without going through it. Holographic imaging and other "new" therapies often get a lot of press simply because they are new. This particular one may be helpful for some people—I am not qualified to judge—but it didn't help Jenny. It's not the type of therapy that matters here but rather how to know if you are in good professional hands.

We entrust to our therapist such fragile feelings that any betrayal of these would be deeply hurtful. The therapist we choose must be worthy of our trust. They must have a professional understanding and an empathetic heart so that, to the extent possible, they can sense where we are along our journey to the other side, which is a place of safety and trust.

Professional credentials from an accreditation-granting body are the best we can hope for to protect us from charlatans—but such a certificate is not a guarantee. Jenny's experience raises awareness to some of the risks entailed in placing ourselves in professional hands. Someone in such dire need of relief has impaired judgment and may be ill-equipped to sniff out dubious claims. This is all the more reason they need only the most *trustworthy* professional making such a referral. Her experience highlights therapy techniques that override our defenses and try to jump-start dimensions of ourselves that have broken down under the stresses placed on them. In Jenny's case, ever intrepid, she regrouped and forged ahead.

Beth

Even as a psychotherapist who is in therapy herself, Beth said it has been surprisingly difficult for her to accept herself as a capable and good person. She holds on to a "distorted, hurtful version" of herself. Through her training and experience, she is aware that people have varying degrees of wanting to know and understand themselves more deeply. She tends to see herself as "in process" rather than "not cured," and she wanted to make clear why she stopped treatment with her first therapist.

"It would be important to talk about why I stopped the first time. I have some very specific reasons. I stopped therapy because there were a series of ways that my therapist let me down. They were traumatic *for me*. They were hurtful and embarrassing to me, but they were nothing major—just normal times where she wasn't as attentive, or times when she didn't say something that I wanted her to say. She wasn't perfect. But it was hard. The final straw—and it brings me a lot of shame because I still think I somehow caused it, my own issues, and all that—was that she would start to nod off. Her eyes would kind of flutter and droop, and she would nod off. I was mortified. That tapped into my own issues: 'I'm sucking the life out of her, I'm draining her, I'm too demanding, I'm too greedy.'

"I know another person whose therapist fell asleep, and this friend was outraged. He chewed him out: 'How dare you!'—where I felt shame and embarrassment. He reacted according to him; I reacted according to me. After that happened several times—and I found myself accommodating, because I wasn't really sure what was going on, but I knew something was going on—'How do I ask about something that I'm feeling so embarrassed about?' It happened a few times, this nodding, bobbing head thing, and I did ask her at one point, I commented not if she was sleepy—I commented very concretely, 'Your eyes are drooping.' She said she felt awake and was not tired. I, of course, could not talk about it anymore because I was so embarrassed, and she didn't, for whatever reason.

"If we ever needed to cancel and reschedule an appointment, I was very aware of, 'Okay, I don't want to go too late in the day because what if she's tired. I'd better go in the morning when in theory people are waking up,' and I thought, 'This is just goofy.' I ended up not coming as much. Around that same time my father was very ill. I wasn't able to see her on a regular basis, and that was my 'out.'

"My experiences in therapy help remind me how difficult it is to sit on the other side. When people come to see me, it's filled with all kinds of meaning, just as when I come to see my therapist, it's filled with meaning. People have all kinds of personal reactions to the process, to the therapy, to the therapist, just as I do. When people wait in the waiting room, I'm reminded of what it's like for me when I'm sitting in the waiting room, and how things that you would think are no big deal, mean something.

"For example, there was a light bulb that was burned out for several weeks above the waiting area, and it reminded one of my patients of her workplace where people aren't responsive and lights are burned out all the time. Nobody is doing what they're supposed to, and she's feeling like she's floundering. So she comes here, and here is this light bulb burned out, and it had a lot of meaning to her. More than just a light bulb. I appreciate that because of my training, but I also appreciate that because of my experience, just as in my therapy when I'm in a session, and there is somebody cleaning the office. We hear this person cleaning, and at times I feel intruded upon, or somebody is around—it's just a person who is cleaning—but it's not. Being in therapy has helped me remain aware that things are significant to people in ways they might not mention or be aware of. It helps me to be a more sensitive clinician.

"Whatever I'm working on in therapy affects my relationships. I'm learning about things, exploring, and remembering things. I'm remembering things I want to forget! How could it not affect my relationships? It makes me more confident or self-assured in some of my relationships. Through exploring and talking about things, I realize more that I can trust my judgment and perception. If there is a dynamic happening in a relationship that I'm in, my tendency is to say, 'Oh, that didn't happen,' or 'They didn't mean it like that,' or 'I'm making a big deal out of it,' or 'I'm overreacting.' By talking about things and coming to some realizations, I see, 'No, you don't have to blame yourself. No, these were your reactions and your perceptions, and you're accurate on that,' so, I guess, calling things for what they are. I have not ended any relationships since I've been in therapy. I do things differently, set different limits, maybe.

"At this point in my life, I don't want to be particularly involved with people where my needs aren't met, or I'm not taken seriously, or where I'm hurt. On the one hand, while I haven't ended relationships, on the other hand, I've *limited* the relationship to where it's not as unhealthy. Maybe I've ended certain aspects of the relationship to bring it more in line where I'm taking care of myself."

Becoming Well

Beth highlighted two important points about the relationship with a therapist. One is how difficult it can be to bring up an issue that has come between patient and therapist. She gave the example of a man who chewed out his therapist for falling asleep; perhaps he grew up in a family where he was allowed to have a voice about what was happening to him. Not everyone did. For Beth, speaking directly with her first therapist about a similar issue entailed feelings of shame and embarrassment.

An experienced therapist isn't threatened by such revelations and confrontations. They are trained, or should be, to help us accept the uncomfortable feelings that can accompany such conversations. By working through a crisis in the relationship with our therapist, we learn how to work through crises in relationships outside their office, strengthening all of those relationships, instead of sweeping under the rug the various issues as they inevitably arise. The relationship with our therapist becomes a model for other relationships in our lives. By mentioning whatever is difficult to say, we reveal something in our makeup; and this can take us on a path to discover a larger issue that may impair our interactions with others.

When we leave a session, or leave therapy, we step back into our everyday lives and into the sense of reality that world imparts. When there is a productive treatment relationship, our therapist becomes central in our lives. We feel the presence of that unique relationship as we go about day-to-day living. We began our lives with the need for a crucial, central relationship; it is what some of us need as adults if we are ever to make ourselves whole again after parts of us were blasted away.

It isn't that our family or friends recede into some middle distance while we take up with this new person, but rather that we come to experience a unique relationship, for we relate to this person on another level of our being. The therapist connects with us on this other level by means of empathy. They come to understand us by sharing in our feelings, accompanying us to places in our emotional memory, and helping us to see in ways we never could before. Few feelings in life can compare to the feeling of being understood, and it is all because of empathy—that essential quality in a good therapist.

Nancy McWilliams writes, "The shortest route to empathy with someone in the role of patient is to take that role oneself. When I first went to an analyst's office, I was shocked to notice that despite my conscious embrace of the idea that there is no shame in seeing a therapist, I was hoping that nobody had seen me go in his door. No amount of intellectual facility prepares us for the sense of vulnerability and exposure that accompanies the role of the help seeker. Nor can we appreciate vicariously the nature of the sense of dependency, in both its positive and negative aspects, that simply comes with the territory of being a client. Adopting the patient role provides the best basis we can have for empathy, even when our own central dynamics are substantially different from those that one of our clients needs to address. And it is the best prophylaxis against contempt."[35] Her observations offer deeper insight into why it is hard to see a therapist, even when rationally we know there is no shame in it. If we don't judge others harshly for seeking professional help, why do we not treat ourselves with the same compassion?

A relationship with a therapist can make it possible for us, in time, to understand and forgive ourselves. One of the most powerful outcomes of therapy is that, in the process of feeling at last that we are understood, we come not only to understand ourselves but to understand others as well. By being understood, a door has opened to the incomparable gift of empathy. When that happens, I believe we are on our way to becoming well.

Summing Up

Therapy affects our relationships—the one we have with ourselves above all. By entering therapy we open ourselves to possibility: of healing, of forgiveness, of deeper self-knowledge and relationships in which we learn to communicate our feelings to others, especially those we love.

For those I spoke with, therapy brought clarity in relationships with family members, friends, and work. How few people in our lives deeply listened to us, with understanding, without judgment or advice, without preempting what we wanted to say, simply letting us talk to hear ourselves think aloud and as we tried to work something out; in therapy some of us could. On the periphery of these conversations were questions of faith, of letting others know we are in treatment, and whether a therapist has struck any "wrong notes."

Therapy moves us into periods of transition in the ways we conduct our lives. We look beneath the surface at subtle currents to help us understand emotional forces at work. We are allowed to tell someone what has happened to us, how things got to be as they are. As we talk and remember, our understanding of aspects of our lives, shapeless in the crush and whirl of daily life outside the therapist's office, become more substantial. We often don't recognize depression and other symptoms when they appear in disguise, but they interfere in the quality of our lives and in our relationships whether we realize it or not. Each of us has to decide whether or not to let anyone know we are in therapy.

Therapy helps us understand the complex dynamics of interactions. It helps us understand the ways the families of our childhood shaped us, especially when their customs contributed to problems for us as adults. Fortified with these insights we look at ourselves more objectively to bring relief and improvement to our lives. By the connection to our therapist we learn how to relate better to others.

In therapy some of us become free of a parent's persistent hold over our lives so as to be no longer bound in service to their needs. Given the complexity of families, the subject of forgiveness is complicated and personal. Offering someone forgiveness before we have explored our feelings, whether in therapy or not, does not necessarily bring the peace we long for. Sometimes talking about it with someone, not just once but over a period of time, helps us come to terms with many deeper dimensions of a difficult matter. Even so, some people became more distant from family members or found new friends.

A good therapy helps us to become more empathic. We learn to recognize when we are in a relationship with people whose development of empathy was stunted, and see how this capacity enriches or diminishes relationships and lives.

In the next chapter we explore questions about the cost of therapy and mental health—the cost of doing nothing or doing something, such as embarking on a journey to know ourselves.

Chapter VI

Weighing the Costs of Doing Nothing, of Doing Something

The burden of mental illness on health and productivity in the United States and throughout the world has long been profoundly underestimated.

—*Mental Health: A Report of the Surgeon* General[36]

THE cost of doing nothing about emotional problems won't appear in numbers alone; the cost is multi-layered, multi-faceted. Research studies enumerate the indirect costs of poor mental health to a society—lost employment, reduced productivity, criminal activity, auto accidents due to mental and substance abuse disorders—but such abstract lists drift toward being meaningless. Most of us don't relate to the societal problem of the "gang activity of fatherless boys." But if you sit beside one such boy, now incarcerated like his father, and he begins to tell about the sorrows of his young life—the poverty, violence, terror—the problem is no longer remote.

Clinicians and clergy, who hear people's sad and painful stories every day, would have a better grasp than the statisticians of the cost to a family of untreated emotional problems. Those who suffer with them, who try to wrestle them to the mat, find the feelings hard to pin down exactly. The cost of therapy—all too easy to quantify—is an inglorious prospect whose outcome, as seen from the front end, is vague and uncertain. It is far easier to go in search of distractions than to look for a therapist or find a way to pay for it.

Hidden costs of untreated emotional problems may take years and generations to unfold. One such cost is peculiarly elusive because it has to do with our defenses. These keep our own emotional problems invisible to us while those of others may be readily apparent. Another defense, used by some more than others, is a tendency to intellectualize emotional problems rather than to feel them. A person may speak fluently in the language of healing and pain, yet nothing ever changes *within* them nor in what they are able to feel.

We don't know the price we pay until blocked emotional pathways have been opened and we are able to feel life fully once again. Then we realize how much we have missed.

Doing Nothing

For a sense of individual suffering I returned to what my interview respondents told me about their lives before they went into therapy, what they saw as if in a rearview mirror. One described "a whole lot of bottled up emotion… a flood of emotion," at the same time being unable to utter a single word. Another said, "No matter what situation in my life came up, I didn't feel good about the way I handled it or what I thought of myself." Others mentioned serious and deep depression, being suicidal, having massive anger, feelings of hopelessness and self-loathing, shame, cutting, and purging.

One said "fear keeps me from a lot of things," another did not want to admit to having a problem, yet another to having "bad self-esteem" (but enough to ask for help). One person described feeling incompetent at work, overwhelmed, struggling, and uncertain, with "horrible sleeping problems and racing thoughts." Another spoke of the pervasive need in her life to take care of her mother; as long as she was compliant in their relationship, all was well between them. There was mention of serious physical problems, feeling responsible for an illness that was somehow incomprehensible, of being unable to "get rid of the grief" for a parent who had died. For some there were failed attempts at suicide. For one person it was being depressed, painfully shy, and afraid of being found crazy. Others mentioned being too insecure to get a decent job, having several run-ins with friends, feeling down all the time and not being able to get much done, overwhelming feelings of terror and anxiety. Another said it was very hard to have any sense of calm. Also mentioned were episodes of mental blackouts, an underlying feeling that something was the matter with her, being unable to see herself as a person separate from her mother, and having a series of disastrous relationships with men. Another described being severely depressed and severely miserable. Still another told of having to go into the men's room to vomit, the panic was so debilitating. One person spoke of feeling like "everybody's rag doll," having no core in a life that "was falling apart." These are all costs recalled in hindsight.

Another cost of doing nothing is that we may become unresponsive to our children's needs or those of others we care about or are responsible for, tending to say and do hurtful things without realizing it. Authority figures, such as bosses, can be notoriously insensitive. Though it's also true that many of us ascribe to them more malicious intent than they deserve. To live and work and love under these strained conditions is more difficult, and all of our relationships are affected (whether we realize it or not). The effects of maternal depression on children are particular cause for concern, well beyond postpartum depression.

> The potential impacts of postpartum depression on a child include depression, anxiety, and attention deficit. Children of depressed mothers may perform more poorly in school and may experience lifelong deficits in coping and interpersonal skills...
>
> In general, however, depressed mothers tend to be less able to read their babies' cues than are non-depressed mothers, resulting in decreased awareness of their babies' needs. Coupled with this behavior is the reduced ability to communicate a range of emotions, making the mother less responsive to her baby. These behaviors usually result in reduced care and stimulation for the baby, although in some instances, depressed mothers who misread their infants' cues may over-stimulate their babies.
>
> Mothers who are depressed tend to engage in less interactive behavior and lack empathy as compared to their non-depressed counterparts; depressed mothers are less likely to read, sing songs, or tell stories to their children.
>
> Maternal depression also affects the physical and emotional well-being of the offspring. The condition often promotes long-term consequences such as a failure to thrive and grow; emotional, behavioral, and cognitive problems; and a lifelong decreased ability to handle stress. Data suggest that children of depressed mothers may have difficulty developing a trusting relationship, therefore impeding subsequent social and emotional development.[37]

Some emotional problems and limitations are strictly private; others show up in marital discord, frustrated career aspirations, meaningless and damaging relationships, alcoholism and addictions, suicides, deepening debt, a pattern of unfinished projects, and family unhappiness. I didn't interview anyone who "did nothing" to change or come to terms with their emotional fault lines; perhaps how well they succeeded in therapy is for you, the reader, to decide, even though none of us is privy to all the layers and facets of anyone's life.

Doing Something by Seeking Help

The cost of doing something about emotional problems entails more than simply time and money. It means limits on spending, possibly a withdrawal from relationships (temporarily or permanently), not having as much time or energy to participate in community activities, the possibility of staying longer in a job or career in order to meet financial obligations. And for many it means dealing with an ever-present sense of stigma; maybe that is another reason some try to "finish" therapy as quickly as possible. Then, on the subject of medication, my interview participants' feelings tended to be as conflict-ridden, stigmatized, and as fraught with worry as the idea of therapy itself.

The irony is that we are unaware of the degree to which a jumbled inner life spills into other parts of our lives. We can't imagine the benefits of airing and organizing our emotions, nor the comfort of sitting on an emotional cushion of just the right medication as long as we need it. These are themes explored in the costs of doing nothing or doing something.

NIMH Economic Costs of Mental Illness

According to the World Economic Forum, the economic health of both developing and developed nations will depend on controlling the staggering growth in costs from non-communicable diseases. The unmistakable message from this report is that mental illnesses are the largest single driver to these costs...Mental health researchers, clinicians, and advocates from around the world...clearly recognized many of the complexities of the frequent chronicity of mental disorders and their interplay with other chronic diseases.[38]

Sarah

Sarah talks about the costs of therapy and her feelings about antidepressants. "Therapy gets real expensive, even though insurance covers some of it.

The financial aspect has always been a struggle because at one point I felt that I needed it weekly, and it was very expensive. I never had a problem with insurance—they always seemed to cover a portion of it. No employer has ever asked, and I've never told anybody.

"Every counselor wanted me on depression medication. I didn't always agree with that. I didn't feel I was that depressed where I needed it. I wasn't crying all the time or couldn't get out of bed. I was functioning. I wanted to go through what I wanted to go through naturally. But I did go on an antidepressant, low doses. I didn't stay on it long. I never wanted to be on it, and I hope to never be on it. I don't think drugs are the answer. I believe people need them, but for me, I can find other ways to deal with my problems. I haven't experienced depression in quite awhile. I do feel down sometimes, but I think it's normal. If I started feeling that way again, I'd go right back into counseling. That would be my first thing."

Gathering Inner Resources

Although therapists have recommended anti-depressants to Sarah, she prefers to put her stock in therapy. A sufficiency of inner resources seems to characterize the mindset of people who turn to therapy for help with their problems—maybe it's an open-mindedness, a learning spirit, and longing for relief. My respondents let me in on the deliberation between not wanting to go and doing it anyway. They were not without reluctance or even something stronger, like resistance, but they found a way to gather their resources. It helped to climb outside of themselves briefly for a different perspective, recognizing that the obstacles outside are no more real than those within. They could even go one step further and admit that things in their lives were not going as they wished, that their lives were becoming more limited, even bringing them toward a breaking point.

This is not far-fetched when we think about those who take their lives rather than draw on their store of emotional wherewithal to find a way to continue living. Therapy sometimes entails overriding the stigma, resistance, a sense of not needing help—that is, our defenses. It means putting those feelings in the back seat, telling them to stay there, and getting on with the work that needs to be done.

That is not saying that people who won't go to therapy have closed minds—nor that everyone who has been in therapy is open-minded—but only to highlight a few necessary ingredients. Among my interviewees these include a willingness to consider their lives from another person's point of view, to let someone else share the burden of their sorrows and defeats.

It is not hard to see ways these lives improved—at least in enough ways to make therapy worth the time and money, often in proportion to their investment; and for some, much more than that. Finding a way to see a therapist is, for some of us, as much about gathering the inner resolve as it is about the money.

NIMH Indirect Costs of Serious Mental Illness

Indirect costs include public expenditures for disability support and lost earnings among people with serious mental illness...The National Institute of Mental Health (NIMH) conservatively estimates the total costs associated with serious mental illness, those disorders that are severely debilitating and affect about 6 percent of the adult population, to be in excess of $300 billion per year.[39]

Hank

Hank replies to my questions about the cost of therapy and about taking medication: "I have issues with money. I'm a big saver. It's very hard, so the money thing does kind of bother me. I know up front that it's better to spend the money to make yourself feel better and to make things right in your life, but I still have a hard time spending the money to do it. But the time? No. All the time is worth it."

Though he had some insurance coverage for therapy, he recognizes that it might be harder for insurance companies to pin down the costs for mental health coverage.

The second counselor Hank saw recommended he ask his primary care physician for a prescription for an antidepressant. "The first time I went to get the prescription it was a little embarrassing, but I just had to keep in mind that if there's something broken, you're going to fix it. That's all it is, and it's nothing to be ashamed of. The chemistry in the brain isn't quite right, whatever it is, and you need something to fix it. The antidepressant worked exactly like it was supposed to. I remember the first day I was on it, something at work happened, and these people are saying, 'Hank! This is happening, and this is happening!' and I say, 'Okay, what's the big deal?' I could see a big change right away, and then it sort of tapered off, and I hardly noticed it. The counselor said that's exactly how it's supposed to work for you. I was on it for a little while, and it seemed to help."

Debating Medication and/or Therapy

Sometimes people look at medication and therapy as separate options instead of each boosting the other's efficacy; sometimes, if therapy is out of the question, medication may be the only option. One woman who declined to be interviewed nonetheless wrote a poignant reply to my request. Her husband had committed suicide three years earlier. She could not revisit that part of her life again, and wrote instead:

> Medications have done tremendous things for people suffering from mental illness, but they need to be taken in combination with extensive, skilled therapy. Often, people prefer to simply take the drugs than to go through the long, painful process of serious behavioral change. My husband was one of those people. He welcomed the medications that his doctor prescribed, and they helped . . . but only to a degree. He went to a therapist for awhile, mainly because of my prodding. But he soon stopped, saying it was too expensive and a waste of his time. He also had a bit of an anti-authority streak. I never could get him to go back. Looking back now, my greatest regret is that I wasn't more insistent. After his death, I immediately sought the help of a therapist, and her help was immeasurable. I often felt like she was the only one I could talk to honestly about the overwhelming feelings I was having.

This woman saw that medication helped her husband, but, like the rest of us, he had feelings that medication alone couldn't penetrate or alter.

Some people think of medication as a comparable substitute for therapy instead of as an adjunct treatment. Using medication without therapy warrants careful thought. A pill is not going to change our lives in the way we long for, and serious emotional conditions are not like common colds that simply run their course. Pills merely hold us steady and keep those of us who are at risk from sliding into the sea.

Christine

Popularity and academic success seemed at odds in Christine's mind with her secret compulsion to binge and purge in high school. Now, four years or so later, she is comfortable that her good friends and family know she has been in therapy for bulimia and continues to wrestle with it at times.

She seems to know when to have a talk with herself when feelings about bulimia, taking medication, perfectionistic tendencies, or depression make their presence known. She smiled during much of our conversation, speaking freely about her experiences, with occasional spells of weeping at sensitive memories.

"I'm on Prozac. I started that about ten months ago. I think at first I immediately thought of the stigma of antidepressants, and at first I thought, 'I don't need an antidepressant!' But then my common sense overruled, and I thought to myself, 'The psychiatrist thinks you need it—I think the psychiatrist knows more than you! Lots of people are on antidepressants, and there's nothing shameful about needing them.' So I began taking them, and I could tell there was a change. My feelings about it were dodgy, like, 'People will think I'm a nut'—again, like the stigma with counseling, but then I was glad I did it. And, again, the perfection. I thought, 'I don't need medicine—I can just do it on my own.'

"I thought that people who take antidepressants are severely depressed, who just sit in their rooms all day in the dark, and I thought, 'Well, I'm not someone like that, so I don't need it.' But after speaking with the psychiatrist I realized it would be helpful. I saw her for just one visit, a full session. I had done blood work when I first started going to counseling, and they did a full physical with a doctor that specializes in eating disorders to make sure everything was okay, so a psychiatrist at the counseling center already had the blood work results.

"I don't feel any stigma about it at all. I'm glad I take it, and I would recommend it to others. It's helpful. I noticed when I first started it I'm not as compulsive. I didn't have as many compulsive tendencies, like with bingeing. It helped with that, and I think I'm not as depressed. I'll have depressive moments once in awhile, but I don't have those nearly as often now, so it helped with that, too.

"I still feel self-conscious when I go to the pharmacy to pick up my meds. When I fill a prescription I feel a little . . . twinge of self-consciousness.

"When I went to the university health service, therapy was free. But back in high school, my mother paid for it, and I used to feel sort of guilty, 'cause I think my mom had to spend it all out of pocket for each session with my therapist because it was a private practice, and I felt guilty at first, but then I realized that my mother cares more about me than money." Here she wept, then brightened. "And my father was very supportive, too. He also wanted me to get better."

Facing Facts about Medication

No one wants to need medication, especially not psychotropic. We would all rather be fine without it. Side effects can be physiological and emotional, such as stigma. And no one wants to spend the money: some of us don't want to spend any money at all on it, some are reluctant because they feel it's not necessary (if you could just be *strong* enough . . .), and some of us think it might be something that is necessary for *others*, but not for us. Misconceptions about it—depressed people sit in their rooms all day in the dark—contribute to the stigma.

Psychotropic medication is a complex subject that needs to be more widely understood and talked about, especially what is involved in taking medication and what is at stake in not taking it. Misunderstandings about psychotropic medication are as widespread as those about psychotherapy itself. We don't want to need medication any more than we want to need a therapist. Perhaps feelings about therapy and medication are cut from the same cloth. All of us want to be bigger and better than that, and none of us wants to feel we are different from others.

Medication can augment therapy. It may keep us functioning by subduing rage or panic. It may soothe us enough to keep us afloat or help us sleep. It may also sustain us during rough stretches in therapy. And, for some people, therapy can make it possible not to need medication anymore.

Allen

The psychologist Allen saw about his panic attacks suggested he supplement therapy with medication. The strength of these attacks—which seemed to be psychological in origin—could take a physical form, as he said previously, sometimes causing him to retreat to the men's room to vomit. "I never felt my inner stress took a physical form up until these panic attacks. Therapy helped me gain the knowledge that part of it involves some things in the brain chemistry. Up until the time of therapy, it seemed to be something I ought to be able to control."

In one session with a psychiatrist, Allen obtained a prescription for Xanax, an anti-anxiety medication, as "insurance" for emergencies. He was disappointed that therapy hadn't completely cured him of the panic attacks nor of the need for medication. It took some time to accept that he couldn't control his mind the way he wanted. When he feels he is heading toward a panic attack, just one pill helps him stay calm enough to get through it.

Even so, acceptance has not been easy, and as he talked about it he circled back to the issue several times. He takes medication for cholesterol and a minor heart condition without a second thought. "It seemed to me it [taking Xanax] was just demonstrative of further weakness on my part, because it couldn't be solved totally with discussion and therapy and greater knowledge about me."

The cost of therapy was another problem for Allen's practical sensibilities, yet in the course of conversations with the therapist he found himself more willing to pay for it. His resistance to the cost of therapy lessened as he began to feel its benefits.

Coming to Terms with Medication

We can sympathize with Allen, but also see how unnecessary and self-defeating is the blame he puts on himself about needing medication. We are more willing to take medication for physical illness, as we see it, than for psychological conditions or those with a possible emotional origin.

The subject of psychotropic medication holds widely different meanings for people. The cost is both financial and emotional, so we accept and reject—sometimes both at once—even the idea of needing it. Most people keenly feel a stigma about it. Some can't afford the meds they need and want and pay an emotional cost of doing without. Still others reluctantly take something, but want to roll off it as soon as possible. Some don't want to put chemicals into their bodies; others of us know we have no choice. And a few of us are grateful for our meds. So there are many sides to the issue of medication, a scramble of facts and feelings about what it does, why it helps, and why it's hard to come to terms with it.

Even in the small sample of people I spoke with, so many of us had similar feelings about psychotropic medication—fear of dependency and addiction, fear of stigma, fear of putting chemicals into our bodies, fear of resulting side effects, fear of being thought weak, fear of not feeling what we need to feel or of masking our feelings, fear of slowing the process of therapy—yet we didn't have those feelings about medication for thyroid or cholesterol. (Ah, a few of those contradictions we prefer to gloss over.)

Given this emotional overlay, it may be unlikely that knowledge of the facts about medication—that you need to take it like a diabetic needs insulin, that some medication will mask your feelings (though not all of them), that medication doesn't necessarily slow progress in therapy, that your body's chemistry is in better balance when you take it, and so forth—will change people's feelings about it.

When facts about medication are useless in the face of strong feelings about them, there is something else going on. We may not want to accept the fact that we have limitations and needs or that one of our children does. It's possible to reach a level of acceptance so that we don't have to pretend something is true that isn't, but that degree of understanding and acceptance takes time to achieve.

A thoughtful perspective about medication is in this excerpt from Stanley Greenspan's *The Growth of the Mind and the Endangered Origins of Intelligence.* He writes, "Medications should be regarded not as cures for disorders but as a means to make the experiences that foster growth available. Unintegrated, piecemeal approaches, whether pep talks from popular gurus or the most powerful new pills, must not be seen as legitimate therapy. Rather, nourishing the developmental process, not simply normalizing a disturbed individual's behavior, should be the mark of genuinely effective treatment. Moreover, cost-reducing plans such as managed care cannot be allowed to set treatment standards."[40] Even those of us who have come to terms with our need for psychotropic (or any other) medication don't want this deficit in ourselves. We don't want to think it's something we can't lick, but maybe by owning it, we needn't feel diminished by it. In fact, maybe our medication allows us to be a better person than we are without it.

Nora

Several years before she went into therapy, Nora had become depressed in response to the stress of a business she and her husband had started that wasn't working out. At that time her religious faith was sufficient to see her through, but eight years later she turned to therapy. The psychologist Nora saw gave her a very general diagnosis of anxiety disorder. She didn't need medication because therapy helped her sort out the main issue that concerned her, which was the relationship with her daughter.

When I asked about the financial aspect of therapy, she said, "It was not inexpensive. But it was worth it. Very much worth it." Insurance helped with the cost.

Then, about twelve years after she stopped therapy, she faced a new set of personal challenges that caused enough stress that she began taking an antidepressant at the recommendation of her primary care physician. "I decided to take an antidepressant to take the edge off and calm me down, and it helped." As the stress waned, she gradually discontinued it, and sought no further therapy.

For Nora, a combination of faith, therapy, and medication has helped her through a few rough spots in her life. She was fortunate to have the benefit of insurance to lessen the expense of therapy.

Weighing Cost and Money

Cost and money have different meanings for people. We fall along a continuum in terms of both our ability and willingness to pay; they are not necessarily the same. There are those who really can't afford it, but somehow do. There are those who can afford it, but who choose a therapist within terms set out by their insurer—which therapist to see, how many times, and at what percentage of the per session cost. Some choose their therapist through a clinic setting that entails no out-of-pocket expense. Some see therapists who offer a sliding scale fee. Others have no choice but to discontinue therapy as soon as the insurance coverage reaches its limit for the year. Then there are those who, despite the cost and sacrifice (with insurance or without), keep their appointments with the therapist with whom they have already established a relationship. In effect, they refuse to accept either the therapist or the terms assigned by the insurance company. Not everyone has that choice.

Therapy is a privilege that relatively few people in the world can afford. For those who can, the question is mostly not whether to go, but how to make it possible. In time, the sense of financial deprivation is replaced by a sense of progress and accomplishment. Our self-confidence and participation in life expand. We find ways to give back to others, more than if we had not been in treatment.

NIMH Panic Attacks and Disorders

People with panic disorder have sudden and repeated attacks of fear that last for several minutes. Sometimes symptoms may last longer... Panic attacks are characterized by a fear of disaster or of losing control even when there is no real danger. A person may also have a strong physical reaction during a panic attack. It may feel like having a heart attack...Panic disorder often begins in the late teens or early adulthood. More women than men have panic disorder. But not everyone who experiences panic attacks will develop panic disorder.[41]

Melanie

Melanie went into therapy despite the criticism of her family. She was briefly on an antidepressant, but, concerned about dependency, she avoids medication.

"It's been difficult to deal with the financial aspects. I have been having financial problems for the past two years, and so it's been difficult to pay for therapy. I've never had insurance for therapy—I guess I felt that my life would be worse off without it."

Choosing Not to Know

Melanie explains how hard it has been to pay for therapy and her fear of doing without it. Her statement is the hinge on which the decision swings for us all: to go into therapy or not, to stay or leave, to continue or let sleeping dogs lie. It's not like a choice between open heart surgery or not; rather, it's about the kind of life you will have.

Ursula Hegi's *Tearing the Silence* examines the choice between knowing and not knowing. Her interview subjects—fifteen people born in Germany who emigrated to the U.S.—are asked to consider the roles of family members in World War II Germany. Their feelings reveal the horror, grief, and shame that followed them when they left their native country some years after the war. The respondents describe the ways their lives were affected by their parents' complicity, sorrow, or silence about the Holocaust: what they knew or didn't know, what they did or didn't do, and how those experiences flowed years later through their children's adult lives.

Many of them have studied and sought out a deeper understanding of themselves and their families; others have chosen not to know. The reader sees the kinds of people they became, the ways in which their choices affect them, and the extent to which they have come to terms with what happened. It is not a question of whether there is a residue from the experiences of that time, but rather the price of not knowing.

One woman avoids knowing how she feels about her father's role as an SS officer: his desertion from the military; his desertion of her, her brother, their mother; the absence of emotional support from her mother; the rape of her mother by Russian soldiers during the war; her own need for order and a tight schedule; her recurring nightmare.[42] These are a lot of feelings and memories to keep under control. Yet only she can make the decision about what she feels is best for her based on a choice between knowing and not knowing, between having a coherent life narrative and one with significant gaps.

Claire

"The first time that I went to therapy the doctor—because there was a supposed suicide attempt, the doctor was very concerned—he must have been a psychiatrist because he prescribed an antidepressant and a tranquilizer, which made me so sleepy that I just gave up taking them.

"My second therapist said that if I felt I wanted medication he would send me to someone who would prescribe it, but he recommended not taking any. He said that I would feel the benefits of therapy more without it. In retrospect I think he was right because I was so out of touch with my feelings that if I'd medicated on top of it, it would have been even harder for me to get in touch with them.

"I did end up, probably after therapy, taking medication. Despite all my therapy and feeling better about myself, I still suffer from feelings of anxiety, especially when I'm faced with situations or people that remind me of my mother. My doctor believes that anti-anxiety medication will alleviate my migraines, and in fact it has. So it wasn't the therapist prescribing it, it was just a very good doctor.

"Several years into therapy, I was having some severe problems with my back, and my doctor recommended an antidepressant—a very low dosage. It's been shown that it's very good for chronic pain, and I have been on low doses of that ever since. It probably helps with the chronic pain and what I believe is a genetic—as well as reaction to circumstances—tendency toward depression, but I have never suffered depression as dark as I did before I went into therapy. Maybe it wasn't a goal set out in a structured way, but my therapist told me if you go through this process you will never feel as deep a depression as you are in now. When I think about it, maybe that was never spelled out or written down on paper, but it has transpired to be true. I continue to take the anti-anxiety medication and a low dose of antidepressant."

"I'm starting to see studies done now where they prove that *both* therapy and medication work much faster and better for most people, and maybe this is something that will happen in time as people come to realize the benefits of using them in combination.

"I think the health insurance companies are short-sighted in limiting the amount of money or visits that a person can go. They'll pay thousands and thousands of dollars for somebody to have heart surgery probably caused by years of stress dealing with problems that maybe they should have dealt with in therapy, but they won't pay a relatively modest sum for somebody to go and deal with what is at the root of a lot of physical problems."

Understanding the Effects of Childhood Trauma

In a deeply touching memoir about the painful relationship with his father, Irish writer Carlos Gabler describes the effect on him as a child on learning that his parents were divorcing. He would live with his mother and not have to see his father again nor be subject to his routine humiliations. He contemplated how that would feel. His halting, "staccato thoughts lengthened into sentences", and as they did he could feel the release of tension in his lungs as he gulped the air, and finally, breathed normally. From that moment, he said, asthma attacks that had afflicted him as a child never recurred.[43] The story illustrates the close tie between our feelings and our bodies, making the point that they are one and not separate spheres.

Child maltreatment, especially sexual abuse, affects the victim's developing brain. Among the consequences for many children are post-traumatic stress disorder and other serious psychiatric problems.[44] The child is unaware of the impact on the brain and of being emotionally overloaded; evidence is inferred by symptoms of psychological distress. Along with being overwhelmed—stunned—the child is prevented biologically from emotional expression in response to what happened. The memory of it has been flung into the dim reaches of the mind, out of reach of the feelings that should have accompanied what happened, blocking them out of consciousness, and ushering in ways for the physical expression of psychological pain.

But can painful events that happened long ago in childhood lead years later to physical illness? Is it possible to prove connections between *this* and *that*—between stresses in childhood and subsequent physical health problems that occur later? If the precise neurobiological links have yet to be identified, one comprehensive study has so far confirmed a relationship between traumatic events of childhood and serious medical conditions in adulthood.

The study, entitled "Relationship of Childhood Abuse and Household Dysfunction to Many of the Leading Causes of Death in Adults"[45] was published in the *American Journal of Preventive Medicine* in May of 1998. It was based on a collaborative effort of the Centers for Disease Control and Prevention and Kaiser Permanente, a large nonprofit, managed care company in San Diego. The initial phase of the study was designed to investigate the link between childhood maltreatment and adult health and well-being. Nearly ten thousand people completed a confidential survey about adverse childhood experiences; more people were included but many of their surveys were invalid when answers to certain questions were left blank (speaking of stigma, shame, and selective forgetting). Survey data were combined with the results of a thorough physical examination that included medical tests and lifestyle questions about current behaviors such as diet, smoking, level of physical activity, and alcohol use.

As I read about the study, I wondered if the questions, like a sieve, were fine enough to reveal emotionally damaging experiences such as Carlo Gebler describes in his memoir, and those that occur in many families and are airbrushed out of family pictures and memories.

The adverse childhood experiences surveyed included emotional, physical, and/or sexual abuse; emotional neglect; physical neglect; mother treated violently; household substance abuse; household mental illness; parental separation or divorce; and/or an incarcerated household member. Individuals who participated were assigned an "ACE score," adverse childhood experiences converted into a measure of cumulative childhood stress. Some respondents reported only one adverse childhood experience; others reported three or more. The questions pertained to the first eighteen years of life.

I looked closely at the definitions of adverse childhood experiences. Emotional abuse was evaluated in terms of how often a parent or other adult in the home swore at you, insulted you, put you down or acted in a way to make you think you might be physically hurt. Emotional neglect was graded along a scale of whether your family was a source of support, strength, and protection by making you feel loved and special. Physical neglect was assessed in terms of whether there was enough to eat or if a parent's drinking interfered with your having clean clothes and being taken to the doctor. These measures were scored based on the degree of exposure to such conditions.

Although the context and specific childhood experiences varied by family, the blunt wording included a wide range of effects. In a summary of their findings, the short- and long-term effects of stressful childhood experiences were numerous health and social problems. Among them were alcoholism and alcohol abuse, chronic obstructive pulmonary disease (COPD), depression, fetal death, illicit drug use, ischemic heart disease (IHD), liver disease, smoking, suicide attempts, multiple sexual partners, sexually transmitted diseases, and unintended pregnancies. In reviewing the list, imagination suggests the extent and cost of some of these at every level of society: individual, family, community, and nation.

The conclusion stated, "We found a strong graded relationship between the breadth of exposure to abuse or household dysfunction during childhood and multiple risk factors for several of the leading causes of death in adults."[46] Since this phase of the study was completed, the medical status of the baseline subjects is being closely tracked to evaluate the relationship between ACEs, health care use, and causes of death. To treat people across the lifespan for these conditions, many of them chronic, imposes massive health care costs.

Growing evidence suggests a link between physical conditions—alcoholism, heart disease, diabetes, dementia, and others—and their emotional roots. Meanwhile research dollars are funneled into finding differences in brain chemistry or genetic make-up, some neurobiological explanation for psychiatric disorders, rather than something that might have occurred within family relationships. But which came first—the disorder in our minds or events in our family, or events that occurred beyond our control, that we have been unable to come to terms with emotionally? By and large, the emphasis—from U.S. government health policy to TV advertising for pharmaceuticals and programs offered by area hospitals—is on physical health and pharmaceutical solutions while the role of psychological cause receives short shrift. Identifying and proving that connection would be hard to do. Perhaps one day a study will figure out the extent to which psychotherapy slows the progression of chronic illness.

In another example, a study conducted by a neuroscientist in Quebec found a relationship between suicide and childhood abuse. Interviews with family members who confirmed the abuse, and autopsies performed on victims, revealed that the victims' brains had forty per cent fewer receptors for a hormone necessary for an adequate flight-or-fight response, thus rendering the victims less resilient and more sensitive to stress.[47]

Studies of violent gang activities often mention that rival gang members who terrorize neighborhoods with random killings appear to have no remorse for their actions. Knowledge of the lives of these young men reveal that they too have been both witness and victim to serious trauma in their lives to which they, too, are now emotionally numb. When I mention to my therapist that a boy I'm tutoring at a juvenile center seems to be without feeling about an event in his life—losing a brother, being shot, being abandoned or beaten by his father, or the criminal activity that put him in jail—he reminds me that these boys have to feel sorry for *themselves* before they can feel sorry for anyone else.

One of the sad ironies is the extent to which those who are victims of maltreatment and sexual abuse blame themselves—blame *ourselves*—when we are not at fault. We were *children*. Reason struggles to penetrate our souls, making it hard to undo the miserable effects of the past. It is possible, as many of us find, to do it in a relationship with someone who knows how to help us work it out, who is strong and dedicated enough not to abandon us when the road we're on feels treacherous, narrow, and steep.

In summary, the experiences of troubled childhoods reappear in the form of multiple health risks later in life, and the maladies from these experiences range far and wide, with implications at every level of our society. For those who can commit to its rigors, psychotherapy helps greatly to ameliorate these effects.

Claire, knowing the conditions of her childhood were related to chronic back pain and migraines as an adult, addressed the problem from all sides to gain relief. For Jenny, the physical symptoms that haunt her are accompanied by a readiness to blame herself—to be *stronger* so as not to need medication—when insufficient will and resolve are not the problem.

Jenny

Despite the abuses of her family, Jenny seemed at ease talking about her experiences. She spoke directly about her medication for insomnia, nightmares, hypervigilance, anxiety, and depression.

"I resisted taking meds the first time, and I resisted it when I went back after I had my son. Why? Because of the stigma! *I'm not crazy*! Even though I thought I was crazy, I didn't want everyone else to think I was crazy!" She laughs. "The person at work who did the insurance, and the pharmacist, and anyone else. . . I mean, at least for me, when I'm in a state of mind like that, I feel like people can see right through me. So I'm at the pharmacy picking up a drug, well, *everybody* knows it's antidepressants and I'm crazy! And the second time I resisted it because I felt that I was stronger than that, that I shouldn't need it.

"Now I look forward to the day when I don't need them. That said, I'm not rushing to get off of it because I need it right now. I sometimes go to the edge and might dip into that dark hole. It allows me to bounce back out of it a lot faster. I'm probably in a depression right now, but it keeps me functional, functionally depressed, so that I can get out of bed and do things and work. I have days when I don't feel like getting out of bed, and I don't want to go to work, but I do it. And when I'm not on meds, when I'm marinating in things that need to be worked out and am depressed, I sometimes can't even function.

I can't get out of bed. I don't want to do anything. I don't want to see friends, I don't want to talk to anyone. I just want to lay in bed with the covers over my head. But I look forward to a day where I can just be happy-go-lucky and don't need that."

Tracing the Effects of Violence

In an article titled "The Neurodevelopmental Impact of Violence in Childhood,"[48] Bruce Perry writes about the effects of violence and fear on the developing child. I chose this article on the Internet, one of the eighty-nine thousand entries in a search for "brain development + trauma," because I heard him speak on the subject in Chicago years ago. Therapists in private practice, and those who work with troubled youth in schools and prisons, see the effects of violence every day, especially on these students' abilities to learn and relate to others.

But Perry looks at only one aspect. He studies the neurodevelopmental changes to the brain to understand the "devastating cost of violence to the individual child"—and its rippling effect on the family, community, and society:

> The more any neural system is activated, the more it will modify and "build in" the functional capacities associated with that activation. The more someone practices the piano, the more the motor-vestibular neural systems involved in that behavior become "engrained." The more someone is exposed to a second language, the more the neurobiological networks allowing that language to be perceived and spoken will modify. And the more threat related neural systems are activated during development, the more they will become "built in."
>
> In summary, then, exposure to violence activates a set of threat-responses in the child's developing brain; in turn, excess activation of the neural systems involved in the threat responses can alter the developing brain; finally, these alterations may manifest as functional changes in emotional, behavioral and cognitive functioning.[49]

Those who live with the effects of abuse or other severe trauma can be a little more forgiving of a need for medication to keep our inner world right side up. Cumulative exposure on the developing brain results in enduring "impairment in multiple brain structures and functions."[50] Some of us may always be on medication because our developing brains were affected by the conditions of our childhood.

NIMH Post-Traumatic Stress Disorder and Depression

PTSD can occur after a person experiences a terrifying event or ordeal, such as a violent assault, a natural disaster, an accident, terrorism or military combat. People experiencing PTSD are especially prone to having co-existing depression.[51]

Beth

During her first therapy, Beth took an antidepressant. Here she explains how difficult the idea was to accept. She also reflects on the time and money involved in her therapy.

"During my first therapy I did go on an antidepressant. I don't believe my first therapist recommended that to me, and I think that meant a lot to me because it meant she could hang in there with me, as opposed to saying, 'You need medication.' I would have interpreted that as her abandoning me—her not hanging in there with me, 'Let's bring in a pill.' However, I wasn't bedridden. I wasn't suicidal. How well a person is functioning makes a difference. My thing was inner turmoil. But it was a very difficult decision, and I didn't think about it at all again for quite some time until it became clear that I really needed to do something.

"When I went to my regular doctor (I didn't go see a psychiatrist, because if I saw a psychiatrist then that would *really* mean I needed medicine, because that's why I'm seeing a psychiatrist!), so I kind of 'guised' it, and went to my family practitioner. I remember when I had the appointment and came in, and I was fighting back tears because it was such a big thing. It made me laugh because here I am talking about not feeling well, and I'm crying (or trying not to cry), and I thought, 'This woman is going to get the wrong impression, and she's going to hospitalize me!'—not that I literally thought that would happen, but it just seemed kind of ironic and funny. I'm talking about this and feeling like crying—not because I'm feeling bad but because the decision in and of itself was making me cry.

"The first antidepressant I tried made me more anxious, like I could jump out of my skin. Then I found another one that seemed to work just fine and helped with anxiety. I was on it and went off it too soon, went back on, went off again too soon—I think I did it three separate times—and this was over the course of several years, and finally went back on and said, 'All right. Enough of this. Just stay on it. You need it—stay on it!' And I stayed on it for a good year. I don't feel I need it anymore, but if things change and I start to feel that way again, it will be again a tough decision, like, 'Oh . . . I couldn't do this on my own . . . ? I thought I had that handled.'" Her voice was tinged with regret. "It would be a big thing. A letdown. I know rationally that doesn't make sense, but that's how I would feel about it.

"The time I've spent in therapy I feel okay about—money, I feel a little bit, I don't know what the word would be, but I pay out-of-pocket. I didn't want to go through the insurance referral process because I wanted to choose my therapist. The second one provides a limited number of sessions, but I would pay for it regardless."

Beth will soon begin seeing her therapist twice a week. She knows that a big point of their talks will be her difficulty paying for twice-weekly sessions. She admits that she will readily go to a store and buy herself something, but wonders why she doesn't feel the same comfort spending money on therapy. She says she knows the money could be "better spent" saving for retirement or investing—yet also knows that's not true. She knows there is something else going on. "I don't know what it is—but there is something more to it than *that.*"

She laughs as she says that, for now, she deals with it by doing it anyway and trying not to think about it.

Resolving the Issues—or Not

Looking at the insurance issue more broadly, Beth is well aware of the discrepancy between physical and mental health coverage. In her clinical practice she does long-term treatment with patients who are on the one hand functioning but, on the other hand, struggling with the unresolved issues that brought them to therapy. For some, when insurance stops, they stop.

With the clarity of Beth's recollection, it's possible to see once again that, apart from physical side effects, medication has different emotional meanings. She shares her awareness that how she *thinks* about taking an antidepressant is at odds with how she *feels* about it; how she *thinks* about spending money on therapy is at odds with how she *feels* about it. She extends her awareness of conflicting views to her experience with insurers—personal experience and that of patients—that they will pay for a little bit of therapy, but only so much, as if to say, "Unless you need to be institutionalized, you should be able to deal with this." If they never resolve the issues that bring them to therapy, they will be weighed down by the same problems.

NIMH Economic Burden of Mental Illnesses

The Agency for Healthcare Research and Quality, cites a cost of $57.5B in 2006 for mental health care in the U.S., equivalent to the cost of cancer care. But unlike cancer, much of the economic burden of mental illness is not the cost of care, but the loss of income due to unemployment, expenses for social supports, and a range of indirect costs due to a chronic disability that begins early in life.[52]

Summing Up

This chapter considered some of the costs of therapy from the perspectives of doing nothing and doing something. Issues related to cost and money held different meanings for people, particularly when facts and feelings were wide apart.

Research studies about the relationship between emotional problems that stem from childhood trauma and physical health suggest they are more prevalent than most of us realize. The long-term effects of severe trauma illustrate the inseparability of body and mind, especially on a child's developing brain.

The cost of doing nothing about emotional disorders far exceeds the cost of doing something. One of the hidden costs of doing something is the stigma of being in treatment. A sense of shame is further perpetuated when news reports lump people into a category of being "mentally ill." Such a term suggests that some people are free of emotional problems while others are not, as if "a bright line" separates us. Those who admit to areas of emotional uneasiness in their lives have to draw on inner resources to override feelings about stigma—not wanting to go, not wanting to need help—even as we know that therapy is a privilege few people in the world can afford.

Medication, as much as therapy, also holds different meanings. It is another arena where facts collide with feelings. The facts are that medication gives us a boost, keeps us steady on our feet, and smoothes out rough edges. They are especially useful in the face of neurodevelopmental impairments and as a way to augment therapy.

However, most people's feelings about taking psychotropic medication were at odds with the facts: "It means I'm crazy." "I'm weak." I'm ashamed." "I fear becoming dependent or addicted." "I feel resisting means I'm stronger." Medication didn't penetrate or alter our feelings, nor was it a comparable substitute for therapy. Depression and anxiety were still felt beneath a protective layer of medication.

Therapy is a way to come to terms with needing to take medication. Simply telling ourselves to "get over it" isn't enough against a nagging sense of shame. Talking with a therapist about what it means to need meds helped some of us come to terms with the fact that we need them. If we are in denial about the psychological/chemical/neurological/biological conditions that makes us need medication, facts alone are unlikely to change our minds.

Some people were unwilling to pay a single penny out-of-pocket while others did whatever was required to help them feel better. Some people planned therapy around health insurance provisions, but often wanted and needed more treatment than insurance allowed.

Those of us who were able, found ways to take responsibility for our emotional problems. We continued in therapy, often paying for it without benefit of insurance. Those of us who stayed with a therapist for the long term not only accepted the increases in fees over the years but also felt profound gratitude to the person who stayed with us. The monetary cost became small compared to what we received in return.

In Chapter VII, interview participants talk about ways in which they gauge progress in therapy as well as its benefits.

Chapter VII

Gauging Progress and Benefits

The hardest thing to see is what is in front of your eyes.
Johann Wolfgang von Goethe

IN early stages of therapy it's hard to evaluate what is happening—if anything is. Some may feel a connection right away, a certain "rightness," and decide to continue. Even then, things can happen beyond our expectations such that the initial yardstick becomes inadequate. So much of the experience is subjective that the ways of gauging progress are hard to define. Also, because therapy at its best is a gift that keeps giving, we may not fully appreciate the extent of its influence for many years.

Therapy is personal and private. Those close to us may be unaware of the changes taking place, though often those changes are observable. A friend doesn't bristle quite as easily, is less tense, snappish, angry... Changes accrue so gradually, becoming a part of who we are and what we understand, that unless we write them down at the moment something seems different, they are swept along in life's hurrying river.

What follows is a nonscientific but sincere appraisal by the dozen people who shared their feelings about the meaning of therapy in their lives. Some of the benefits and gauges are readily apparent; others are more subtle. Some signs of progress were the ability to be more objective, get beyond blame, find answers in themselves, and hold onto the changes in themselves. They began to accept that some things may or may not work out the way they wished. Some respondents mentioned being able to find emotional truths, learn to work through issues, become more psychologically minded, and understand themselves more deeply.

Gauging Progress

One day I watched children in a preschool as they went about studying the properties of items they had collected—feathers and corks, ribbons and bottle caps, string and paperclips, rice and beans, plastic and wool. With mounting excitement they were learning about the attributes of these things—color, size, texture, toughness or fragility, soft edges or sharp ones, and whether the items would float or sink. Little did they know they were learning to observe, analyze, compare, and classify what they'd found. Their process suggested a way of gauging progress in therapy.

Someday for these children the resulting skills from their explorations will transfer from concrete items to abstract ideas. What they learned will be useful well beyond preschool. Their life experiences and teacher-planned activities, along with—and this is crucial—talking about their observations, helps them incorporate these new ideas and words into an understanding of the world. Meanwhile, their self-confidence builds quietly with each achievement.

Their explorations are similar to how we learn in therapy. Our experience is processed through a filter of language in order to master our feelings and awareness of what's going on within us, blending old stuff with new. We learn to recognize and name feelings, and to own even the ones that are embarrassing, ugly, or painful. In doing so, our confidence grows, along its own timetable, in a process that can't be hurried. For some of us, hurry would create unnecessary anxiety.

Children learn at a faster rate because they don't have to *unlearn* anything. For us, unlearning is a big part of the process, which begins slowly in a developing relationship with another human being who, with our help in the back-and-forth of conversation, tries to understand how we feel and why we have certain problems. In the process we may work through a difficult experience in our lives well enough to find ourselves more or less at peace with it—it no longer frightens, preoccupies, controls, or eats away at us. This is one of the achievements of therapy from which the benefits unfold.

Sarah

Sarah's history in counseling began with her brother's suicide. These are her thoughts as she reflected on therapy's meaning to her.

"Internal stress caused me to overeat and suffer depression. Sometimes I would be thin or overweight. I was always thin in my childhood and teen years, then struggled with weight gain in my later twenties. I think this was due to not feeling what my purpose in life was. I felt lost mainly because of my childhood. I suffered asthma and allergies since childhood, and I know this is from stress and not eating right.

"Through therapy I realized I was smart and talented. When my self-confidence increased, so did the ability to control the weight ups and downs. I also attribute a lot of changes to maturity. It took me awhile to mature since my parents were immature themselves."

She takes herbal medication for asthma and allergies, but no antidepressants. "I feel like a stronger person, and I don't feel so ashamed. I was handling situations in my life in ways that were better. I learned not to take things so personally. In a relationship, that's another story. I'm still working on that."

"Without therapy I don't think I'd be where I am now. What reminds me of that is my brother, because we were a lot alike, and he ended his life because he felt so bad. I feel fortunate that I had help.

"I don't judge people as much anymore. I try to be more compassionate—I've learned that through counseling. I just kind of grew up emotionally. I learned in therapy that I'm not such a bad person. I treat myself better and am not so hard on myself. I used to question everything I did—always thinking that I was wrong or bad. Now I treat myself as I would treat other people. It's nice to live without those feelings."

Becoming Stronger

There are many paths to achieving physical strength. Achieving emotional strength is more complicated, or at least less straightforward. Our ideas differ about what it means to be strong. Each of us has ways in which we wish we could be stronger, less vulnerable to being hurt, better able to be more, or to achieve more. One person's idea is to be less worried about what other people think, which differs from another's about being less sensitive to rejection or criticism or border crossings. Yet another wants to be more disciplined or less subject to fits of depression. Sarah says that since therapy she's not as hard on herself, and adds, "It's nice to live without those feelings."

In certain moods *those* feelings seem to be gone, but do they vanish? Or do we just learn to manage them better? Is it possible that any of us stop being our old selves? Maybe, with deeper self-awareness we become less reflexive, more adept at modifying our responses in keeping with how we want to live our lives. The process entails becoming more objective about ourselves and the important people in our lives.

When we were children, our parents for a time were our whole world—the earth, sun, moon, and stars. They seemed all-knowing, all-powerful, and all-wise, which is why whatever they said and did must have seemed to be what was best for us, for surely they loved us as much as we loved them. But parents are fallible and, if children are allowed, they become more discerning as they mature, able to see a few weak spots in those beloved figures. Even then we can't be objective about them—they're our *parents*. None of us at the time think about our parents' qualities or qualifications, or how our destinies are partially shaped by them—we're *children*.

By talking about our family in therapy we become more independent and objective, and where possible, become closer than we were before. We have the chance to reappraise the situation we grew up in and see how our families helped to make us who we are. That knowledge is confidence and freedom, in a matter of degree.

Knowing our families is an indirect path to knowing ourselves. Stepping back to look at them deepens our self-understanding. It helps us see why we might think of ourselves in ways that may be at odds with who we are and how others see us. Instead of overriding these feelings with motivational slogans, we study how these ideas contribute to self-defeat and disappointment. Then we can begin the hard work of modifying faulty ideas and unwelcome feelings toward strength that is durable and authentic.

Hank

Hank noted, "When you can listen to what the therapist is saying and he kind of makes you think in a different way, he sees things just a little bit differently—that's successful to me.

"Therapy has made me grow a lot. I think you live in a small world if you can see things only from your view, and you're a more difficult person to deal with.

"I'm a manager of blue-collar guys. It's what I started working as, so I understand what makes them tick. From therapy I learned you always try to look at the other person and to look at *their* view. I've had to deal with a lot of conflict between people that work directly together and have to resolve their problems. I put on my counselor hat a lot of times. 'Okay, when he does this, how does that make you feel?' I'm making the other person realize how the other person feels when this happens. I've resolved a lot of conflicts that way.

"In my industry there are very big egos, very stubborn, very narrow-minded people—'It's *this* way, and this is the *only* way!' I try to make people that I work with look at things. If there's a problem, I'm not going to say, 'Don't do things this way anymore.' I'm going to say, 'Hey, this is the way we should be doing it.' I use encouragement to direct people, and I've learned that through counseling. . . . It's opened my eyes, I'd say. A lot. A whole lot. Before counseling I didn't realize the mistakes I was making with my wife. You realize what you may have been doing wrong, why there are problems. I was more frustrated, thinking that I was fine, everything else was wrong.

"And I can kind of counsel my daughter. I try to understand why she's doing what she's doing. I don't think I would have learned anything from my daughter if I hadn't opened my mind a little bit."

Walking in Another's Shoes

The capacity for empathy, its potential present in most people from birth, may be nurtured in us by kindness and understanding, or restricted and snuffed out. Varying degrees of stress during childhood lessen the chance that we will mature emotionally. At its most severe, we don't grow beyond the self-centered world of babies. However charming or charismatic we may be to compensate for what we lack, our world is all about us, preventing us from developing empathy, from recognizing others as separate beings, from feeling joy or wonder or love, or from forming enduring relationships.

Therapy raised Hank's awareness of communication in which issues are resolved and people's needs are addressed. He became more aware of needing to look at issues from another person's point of view and to be wary of hasty judgments and rigid pronouncements. It may keep him from becoming someone who thinks his view is the only one by opening him to consider many possibilities instead of only *this* or *that*, my way or no way.

An awareness of empathy, of those who have it and those who seem to lack it, is another aspect of being psychologically minded. It gives us insight into possible reasons for relationships getting derailed. It also helps us find our way in what can seem an otherwise inexplicable morass of bad feelings. For some of us, therapy is a way to achieve emotional maturation that we missed out on in childhood, including becoming more empathic.

We don't read a book and become empathic. If not in the family, it can happen in a relationship with a caring and skillful therapist as we open ourselves to feelings that were short-circuited by conditions over which we had no control. Empathy is not like a lucky penny in your pocket, something you have or don't. Rather, it is a capacity that may be large or small, and by degrees between.

Christine

"Without therapy," Christine said tearfully, "I think I'd be unhappy, probably would be physically ill from the bulimia. I wouldn't want to go out as much, because I wouldn't want to eat, because then I purge and then feel guilty and stressed out. So I think that's how my life would probably have been.

"One thing that happened right after—and I would say it was as a result of therapy—I met my boyfriend. I wouldn't have had the nerve to talk to this boy because I'd be so shy. But I thought, *Nothing bad is going to happen, just talk to him*. So I did and he asked me for my number later! So I am very proud of that. A good thing came of it. We've been dating almost six months now. He's my first boyfriend, too! Now it's something to smile about—instead of cry."

She thought another moment and then added, "I think my family is more open to therapy for themselves now. My mother is under a lot of stress, and she's talking about going to a counselor for various reasons, and my brother, he's having a drug problem, and he's going to go to a counselor. Maybe I sort of paved the way for other members of my family.

"I'm more pleasant and fun to be around now that I'm not as stressed and worried. I've also gotten closer to my friends after telling them about the counseling. It's something personal that I've shared with them, and they've shared with me. It's a bond between us."

Then I asked her how she gauged progress. "First was stopping the binging and purging. That was the most obvious. Also, becoming more cognizant of my negative inner dialogue—being able to talk to myself more rationally. When I realized I wasn't having as many negative thoughts, and when I did I would catch them, that was progress.

"Therapy has made me healthier and happier, and a lot less stressed out. I have more energy. I went to a dietician, and I'm choosing better foods to eat. I can enjoy eating now and not feel guilty like I used to. I feel better about myself and my body and just happier all around.

"My goals were to stop the binging and purging, and stop being negative, and that's what happened. I was successful in that, pretty much."

Becoming More Self-Aware

One of the benefits Christine highlighted was "becoming more cognizant" of her thinking patterns, of "being able to talk to myself more rationally." Her therapist had lifted one pick-up stick from the scattered pile in her brain, and freed it from the rest. It was one Christine could use.

Success—in therapy and in life—is closely tied to self-awareness. We have to notice when and which of our behaviors cause people to turn away; we have to notice repeating patterns of failed efforts; we have to notice the moment when our mood turns dark because from that point we can re-trace our emotional steps to figure out why. Self-awareness is an active, dynamic process of inquiry, response, and readjustment; a therapist gives it depth and accuracy. Again, it's not a matter of having it or not, but a matter of degree.

Greg

"When you're depressed you don't always realize you are. There is no simple test, so it's something of a problem to tell when you need help. You grow up thinking—however you grew up—that it's perfectly normal, that's how everybody deals with it. It's really hard to judge on your own that you have an issue or you need some help. And likewise it's hard to tell how much better you are. It's kind of up to you and the doctor, or whatever your therapist is, to jointly explore what the problems are, then also jointly figure out how much progress you're making and jointly figure out when to take a break or quit therapy. It's definitely a team effort. It's really hard to judge for yourself on both ends of it—starting or stopping.

"I began to feel more energetic and optimistic and get more done and have good relationships with my family. I probably did observe changes in myself, but it's hard to put your finger on it. It was very distressing to see my mother go downhill. It was never easy to deal with, but with therapy it became less distressing. I guess that's the word. It wasn't quite so distressing. How much of that was due to therapy and how much to just going along over time with it, it's hard to say, but I could deal better with the situation.

"I had an excellent therapist. He was a doctor and came highly recommended, so I didn't have to explore and look for a different approach if this one didn't work. He was very kind, very gentle and accepting, even-keeled. He tried to suggest helpful things for me and my mother, both."

Achieving Collaboration

We are unaware of it at first, but even our early attitude toward our therapist tells something about each of us. Into that space we bring our fears, biases, preconceived judgments, cynicism, and hopes; especially fear and hope.

The relationship may start well enough but in time it becomes more complicated by shadows on the wall. Dim feelings we begin to notice never seem to get hauled to the surface; feelings of dread, superiority, a sense of threat, or longing all have meaning. They may keep us from having a comfortable relationship with the therapist. That's okay; that's one of the indirect goals of therapy.

That relationship with the therapist is the heart of the matter. (If it weren't, a computer would suffice.) Into the space between client and therapist (patient and analyst), we bring our openness, capacity to trust, and willingness to engage; our fears, our need to hide or withhold; our ability to be close and our need for distance; our need to be superior to the therapist or subordinate. When Greg says "jointly," it means together you figure out the problems, evaluate progress, decide to continue, take a break, or end. The ability to collaborate with our therapist is an achievement.

Allen

As we saw earlier, Allen saw a therapist fifteen years ago about his panic attacks. Now, "I can see that things which might have caused me to be panicky, I can get through now without medication. Therapy helped me understand what's going on. I enjoy people too much to be trapped in my house."

He gauged his progress by whether his condition improved. It took some time, but he told himself that change wouldn't happen overnight.

"Has the quality of my life improved? Yes. Have I come to a greater understanding of the factors I'm wrestling with? Yes. Am I more accepting of myself, based on that therapy? Yes. Those are some of the things that I use to measure progress." He said he would like to reach a point where he doesn't feel the need to carry just-in-case medication, but has accepted that maybe that won't happen.

He finds he is able to do things "automatically" without feelings of panic, and when anxiety comes calling, the incidents are fewer.

"My life [before counseling] was good, but not as good as it could have been. It felt like things were closing in on me or that I was avoiding some situations, things I couldn't deal with. Certainly there were some periods of very high anxiety before counseling, and also that business of the unknown—not knowing a lot about what was going on—created fears in me. I sure wrestled with thoughts like 'Am I losing my marbles?' 'Am I going insane—or some version of it?'" he laughs. "And that cropped up a lot before counseling. Other things were going on, but insanity or a nervous breakdown it wasn't. Now, I don't know that I bought it right away just because he [the therapist] was saying it, but in working with him, I came to accept that more.

"The life I led afterwards—and just the greater knowledge—are benefits. From that knowledge about me I was able to work towards accepting some of the things about me as being not bad/not good—that's how I am. Trying to discern what things need to be worked on, that I could work on changing, versus what things I just have to accept as part of who I am. And that's a hard one to call. You can't just say, 'Well, that's how I am, I'm not going to change.' If I can change some things, then the therapy helps me identify some of them.

"Therapy has enabled me to have a quality of life that I wouldn't have had, I'm sure, had I not pursued that. As hard as it was to discuss things and to open up to someone I didn't know—a stranger—maybe that's a good thing. Maybe it's harder to talk to someone you know about these things, but it's been worthwhile."

Being Able to Open Up

The difference between opening up to a therapist and opening to a stranger on the train is that you don't see the stranger again. To open our hearts to a therapist, to talk about our embarrassment, fears, and shame, then return to face that person again and find we are still loved, means a great deal. If Allen had never shared his embarrassment and other concerns, he would have left with the same feelings he had brought when he entered.

It is natural to want to protect sensitive areas. The problem is that the secrets we hide hinder us in relationships. Withholding from our therapist (assuming we feel sufficient trust and respect) suggests that we withhold ourselves from others, remaining aloof and apart, a stranger even to ourselves. Opening up can be the first step to opening ourselves to someone else. If not, we are stuck, missing out on a lot, churning in conflict.

In sharing our pain with someone who understands, we ask that person to bear witness to what we have experienced. The sharing is deeply consoling, in time helping us to heal. We no longer have to bear it alone. For those of us who have experienced a lot of hurt, we must face each instance in our memory. It means going together through layer after layer of protective coating to find the original, authentic material of who we are. It doesn't happen overnight.

Finding a therapist we can talk with in time helps us to be more open to life, not living underground in the dark, squirreling away our treasured acorns. Our therapist's office—and the space between client and therapist—is the laboratory where we learn to locate our feelings and talk about them, where we learn to see and think about ourselves differently, and bring that knowledge and understanding into our relationships in the world outside.

From a therapist we can learn about love: how it feels, how it sounds, what it means. All in words alone in that sanctified space between two people.

Nora

"I'm more confident as a result of therapy because of the way to figure things out if someone has a different perspective. Without therapy my life would have been more frustrating. I was trying to communicate and get along with my daughter, and it just wasn't working. At least I have been more aware of her feelings now so that we can communicate better, or even say, 'I didn't mean to do that.' We probably wouldn't have been as close or as forgiving. But there has to be willingness on the other person's part, too."

Knowing How to Work Things Out

Nora's simple statement holds a truth: "But there has to be willingness on the other person's part, too." Both parties in a dispute, a distancing, or a disappointment must want to heal the rift. People have different tolerances for living with estrangement, loneliness, sorrow, or fear, but I wonder whether some people—even most—don't know how.

We learn how to work things out (or not) in our family. Those who have this particular disability—of not knowing how to heal rifts, how to talk things out, how to resolve differences—may be unaware of its absence. They may take no notice of how subtly it interferes with their lives: not seeing how unhealthy guilt steers their course, not seeing signs of festering resentment, not seeing empty gestures of apology, not seeing a need to distance oneself or to hide.

If bitterness and anger have been swept under the rug, it seems unlikely that sitting down to talk can undo years of ignoring the pain we inflict on each other. Therapy can help people, individually or together, find a way through a morass of judgments and ill will so the bad feelings don't go on forever. If we don't have resolution, then perhaps resignation with peace.

James

James looks at his experience in therapy from a distance of several years, recalling the discrepancy between what he was saying about his situation and what he was doing about it.

"There's a difference between knowing what the problem is and knowing how to do things that are going to help. It's not enough to understand the situation; you sometimes need help figuring out what you're doing that's stopping you from getting there. I remember many times that I would say something, and my therapist would point out that what I'm doing is not consistent with what I say I want to change or improve, so I'm not being honest. If I wanted to help Daniel, and I wanted to help myself, and I'm doing these things—is that really helping? No. Therapy helped me realize that my actions weren't necessarily in line with the way I saw things. They were absolutely at odds.

"I've thought of seeing a therapist again in a different way, not necessarily to address any problem that I'm having, but to just be able to talk to someone and explore issues. That feels very *healthy* to me. I felt then that I was doing something *good.* And some things came out that I didn't even know were going to.

"If I hadn't talked with someone other than family or friends, if I hadn't talked with someone professional who would teach me to bring things out of myself and discover things in the way that it happened, I can't imagine what would have happened. Maybe I would have been fine in a different way. But I think I would have tended to wallow in the sameness because moving ahead would have been hard without the understanding and the work that was involved in therapy."

Finding Emotional Truth

In our haste to be agreeable we sometimes—or always, if it's our default setting—smooth things over and carry on as before, as if what was done or said was acceptable. Or we ignore the depression we feel on waking and check ourselves into a busy, cheerful mode for the day, ignoring our true feelings until they find expression in a headache or an extra drink. When there are layers (on layers) of these accommodations, true feelings can get buried.

Examples of such accommodations are everywhere. Perhaps we don't want to accept that our son has problems at school; the teacher is a jerk. We may not want to face the disruption and agony of divorce, so we sidestep the issues by focusing on all the good things about a spouse, never mind the loneliness and hurtful remarks. We don't want to revisit a troubled time in our life when we were cruel to someone, so rather than finding the courage to talk it out or write a letter of apology, we give ourselves a pass and let someone else carry the blame. We can't bear to admit a parent's failings or risk losing favor with that beloved ideal, so we shift our anger onto someone else. These are familiar domestic scenes that throw emotional balance a little off kilter. In a similar way, our bodies need to be in balance. Repetitive stress on a shoulder takes its toll, though the strain may not show up for years. It may appear as "carpal tunnel" at the wrist, when in fact the strain and tension are at the neck and shoulder. Self-deception in relationships also carries a price; we just don't necessarily know what it is.

When James says, "So I'm not being honest," it's not that he's dishonest. The nature of defenses is to protect us from emotional truths we prefer to avoid. We think we are being honest with ourselves, but don't realize the ways in which we obscure and distort how we really feel. A therapist's objectivity brings needed support in becoming more emotionally honest; we can be honest with ourselves and with others without being brutal.

NIMH Response to Trauma

[In recent years], the United States has experienced a series of manmade and natural disasters. Large numbers of people in this country have been exposed to potentially traumatic events...Most survivors have intense feelings after a traumatic event but recover from the trauma; others have more difficulty recovering especially those who have had previous traumatic experiences, who are faced with ongoing stress, or who lack support from friends and family and will need additional help.[53]

Melanie

Melanie said, "The way I gauge progress is when I handle a situation in a better way than I did before. In the first therapy it was the whole idea that I could make a living, save money, and have a household. But now it's more that I handled a situation well. When I run into people stepping on my boundaries, previously I might have yelled or screamed at them. I realized that those people would villainize me for yelling at them, never realizing that they had stepped on my boundaries.

"More recently I waited a few days. I lost that need to take care of it right away. I sit on it, and I think about it, and then I pick a moment to talk to those people and say, 'Listen, I have a problem; this is something I don't expect from you, and you walked on my boundaries.' They say they're sorry—but then they always try to turn it around against you! I just say, 'Well, thank you; I wanted to tell you this, but I've got to go now' and didn't listen to the rest of that conversation. I was really proud of how I handled that. I'm still in contact with these people—of course they're not my best friends—but because of handling the situation in a different way, I'm setting clearer boundaries, which I don't think I ever had before. I would just get mad.

"Also, I'm starting to be a little bit more accepting of other people's different ideas and looking at subtle ways that people are different and being less concerned about how it affects me. I'm no longer looking at the world only from my point of view.

"Anytime you learn something, you're going to have periods of growth and then a plateau. Because not only after a period of growth are you tired, but you need to fully assimilate that growth. What you learned previously is becoming a bigger part of who you are.

"It's sometimes hard to determine whether you're at a plateau or an impasse. I don't know how to figure that out. Maybe if you're at a plateau for a year, you should think about seeing a different therapist. That was one of the problems with my first therapy. I didn't move up for quite awhile, and when I started discussing what other things we could do, it became traumatic for my therapist. There wasn't an open exchange. I started looking at what else I could do to *move up*—other activities or classes or meditation—and she wasn't supportive. She got defensive, and that should have been my clue that there was a problem.

"In therapy I learned that I have a huge amount of guilt and extremely low self-esteem. I learned that I have good intentions and some unkind. I learned who I was, because I didn't have any knowledge of who I was before therapy. In fact, I only knew what I didn't like—I didn't even know how to say what I did like! It's been a difficult road because I was not really raised to have an identity of my own. What I've gained is some identity, some autonomy, some ability to say, 'I like this, and I like that, I enjoy this, and I enjoy that, and that I want this or that.'

"The benefit of psychotherapy for me is I've been able to have a life of my own instead of one that was attached to my mother and her needs. It was debilitating for me, and I have a freer life now. Without therapy I would probably be living with my parents. I wouldn't have a life if I didn't have therapy."

Having Less Baggage

Baggage, that stuff from the past, weighs us down and interferes with self-esteem, work, and relationships. Unexamined matters get in the way of seeing clearly, even causing us to take things personally or shoot ourselves in the foot. Therapy is where we open those old, worn valises, sort, stash, and sometimes let the contents go.

Melanie says she is learning to handle situations better; to distinguish between a genuine apology and self-justification in the guise of one; to make her needs clear without losing either her dignity or a friend; to discern between friends she can be close to and those she can't; to realize that her parents won't change, yet still be clear about her needs; and to differentiate between her issues and someone else's so she is less inclined to take things personally.

Every time she said, "I'm starting to realize," that was progress. When she began to see that people were behaving as they were because of their own issues, that was progress. When she found more polite ways to ask people to respect her boundaries, that was progress, too. When she learned to recognize and say what she liked (and didn't), that was progress. And when she began to see that her therapist seemed to be unwilling to let her augment their work together with meditation or a class—that also was progress.

Sometimes people imagine they're going to become dependent on their therapist in an unhealthy way, but when Melanie began to feel constrained by her therapist, she realized it was time to leave. It must have been painful to feel let down by someone in whom she had placed her trust, and I wondered whether she didn't feel twinges of guilt about leaving. I suspect it would have been hard to leave—with a history of feeling responsible for her mother's well-being—perhaps feeling she was hurting her therapist.

The situation illustrates why therapists need to have done work on their own issues so they are less apt to impose their needs onto their clients. It also suggests how glorious a feeling it is even to *begin* to learn how to differentiate what is your issue from what is the other person's. That Melanie, along the way toward making other changes in her life, could sort through her feelings and opt for her own best interest seemed impressive progress to me. I wanted to hand her a bouquet and ask her to take a bow.

Claire

Claire noted, "It's not a linear process, that's for sure. There were times when I was able to express either extreme grief or extreme anger, and I felt such tremendous relief and peace afterwards that that was a sign of progress, that I had dealt with something I had blocked. I got it out in the open. And certainly I started feeling more . . . not that I ever wanted to die, but that I wanted to live rather than just exist.

"It was progress to me that when people treated me in a way that was unacceptable I was able to let them know, which was something that I *never* could have done [before therapy]. It was not so much progress as a series of small victories. I would achieve one of these things . . . that I stood up to somebody! Before, if somebody was mean to me, I would back down and slide into a corner or cry. When I actually stood up to them, I'd tell my psychologist, and he'd praise me and metaphorically pat me on the back, so progress happened in that kind of way.

"It was never in the way that somebody learning to play a musical instrument gets better and better. It was a big thing to be able to stand up to somebody, when I had been like a little mouse before.

"If I hadn't had psychotherapy I don't know where I would have ended up. Being in touch with my feelings, being able to set boundaries, being able to stand up for myself, being able to choose my relationships with more care and not just having relationships—and I'm not just talking about sexual relationships—I'm talking about all kinds of relationships. If I knew someone and we got friendly, I always felt that I had to have a relationship with them, and I learned that some of them were not healthy or were not good for me. I did a lot of weeding out of those kinds of relationships. My life became much more about what was right for me to live my life in a way that I was happy—for me.

"Maybe somebody else's ideal might be to be married and have children, but I like living on my own. I like being single. I have the freedom to choose and do what I want, and I think all of those things—setting boundaries, deciding what I wanted in my life and from my life—spring from the therapist asking me, 'What do you want in your life?' For the most part I can't say that I know what I want for a career, but that's a whole other issue. But if I didn't have to work to earn a living, I know what I enjoy doing. I was not in touch with that before.

"What I've learned, too, is that I was afraid of not pleasing people or saying what I felt. I thought people wouldn't like me if I did. I've learned that people respect me a whole lot more when I speak my mind. I am who I am, instead of pretending to be somebody that I think they want me to be. I'm very much more living in my own skin, being myself. I don't think I would willingly go along with something I did not want to do, as I so easily did before, and then be unhappy about it.

"Before, I never thought that I had the right to live for myself, to please myself. I think that's one of the biggest changes. Now when I do something I think about 'Is this right for me?' Growing up with the mother that I did I always had to think about what *she* wanted. It's okay to do what is right for me and what I want for me.

"When I entered therapy I was in such a deep, dark place that I didn't even know what a goal should be. I didn't know what it was to be a happy person or to be what I am today. I might answer that question very differently had I gone into therapy at this stage of my life. Certainly I'm out of the deep, dark place I was in; I'm not having the terrible depressions. . . . I mean, at the beginning of therapy, I definitely wasn't able to have a goal for therapy other than wanting to go on living—and I definitely want to go on living for a long time."

Finding a Way Out of Depression

Depression obscures the view of a way out. Other people seem to go about their lives with purpose and verve, while we move around as if under water, every movement difficult, frustration intense, therapy (seemingly) interminable, all feeling strangled by depression, and hope barely alive.

Some people think depression is about adjusting your attitude; or that by reading a self-help book you will learn what you've been doing wrong all these years and will get out from under that dark cloud. That's neither what depression is nor how to find relief. Antidepressants can help, but therapy with a good therapist is better yet. We learn our depression is not a matter of personal failure. Each episode leads to the interior of ourselves where we find feelings that have been held back.

When we begin to feel something, it's like the arrival of spring to bleak and frozen tundra.

I love the following observations Nancy McWilliams makes based on her work with clients: "Very often, the kind of change that the client originally envisioned is not the kind that occurs, only because what does occur is something the client could not have initially imagined. To move into areas that are emotionally new, the client must proceed on a kind of borrowed faith. If the practitioner proceeds with integrity, the client will eventually feel trust in the therapist as a person; the therapist, meanwhile, exemplifies faith in the client, the partnership, and the process. A woman coming to treatment may want to learn how to relieve a depression and instead learns to express previously unformulated feelings, to negotiate for herself in relationships, to identify the situations in which she is likely to feel depressed, to understand the connections between those situations and her unique history, to appreciate her tendency to blame herself for things that are outside her control, to take control over things that had previously seemed impervious to her influence, and to comfort herself instead of berating herself when she is upset. As the therapeutic process evolves, she gradually loses all the vegetative, affective, and cognitive symptoms of depressive illness. But more important, even though before the therapy she may have enjoyed long periods of freedom from diagnosable clinical depression and thus could conceive of feeling better, she could not have imagined the depth of authentic feeling that is now becoming a reliable feature of her emotional landscape."[54]

In conversations with a therapist, what had been a wordless, amorphous mass takes on a form of words, ideas, insight, even humor, its outline at first vague and tentative, then more alive. This takes time to unfold because we have our reasons for constricting our feelings.

Those whose emotional problems were debilitating enough to drive us into treatment are, in some ways, fortunate because of it. People who are able to "function just fine," yet who struggle with issues they shove aside, also struggle. The years slip by and they continue to live with their assorted problems, none of them serious enough to drive them into therapy. Or if they do go, it's with a half-hearted effort for a short time. They aren't desperate enough—or haven't imagined the possibilities. Therapy's gifts don't just happen during pleasant chats; they are the result of hard, sometimes harrowing emotional work.

That's why those of us who are driven into therapy by the size of our problems—and stay there till the job is done—are in so many ways the lucky ones.

Rose

"When I look back at the progress I've made in my social life and in my work, I don't think I would be as successful as I am in my field if I didn't know how to listen like I do. It has to do with having been listened to and hearing yourself talk. You have to hear yourself. Also, I probably have a little bit more courage than I did as a kid. I would never just go jump in a lake without knowing how cold the temperature is, so I'm a little more of a risk taker now than I would have been.

"Some of the progress might be because of aging, but I'm more willing to take a stand on things. I have more confidence in my own ideas than I did before. I was always looking to other people to feed them to me, and then perhaps I would reject something I didn't want, but I don't know that I really had my own ideas very much. I let my first husband rule the day. People looking at us would never have known we were in trouble. I wasn't going to let it show.

"I'm a more empathic person than I was before. I can allow for other people's misfortune, that they too have suffered. When I was growing up I dismissed it. Now I 'get it' about other people, that we all go through life with our struggles. And some things you just can't fix, although one tries.

"One learns to live with ambiguity—and this is another benefit, I think, of psychotherapy. Because you can't really measure time. You can only do it in retrospect. You can say, 'Ah, that period helped me to see this.' So the ability to live with ambiguity is a big benefit, because you have to live in a state of not knowing for so much of the time and still be able to go on with your life. You have a session, and you're in this crazy place, and then you leave, and you have to be in another place.

"I still don't like to make an appointment with anybody after my sessions, so I keep that time for myself. I used to make plans with people *after* my session in order that I wouldn't get much done during the session. It would be a way of avoiding dealing with things.

"In certain ways I don't tolerate as much as I used to. In ways I am much more protective of my time, whereas before I never would have done that. Not in a million years would I have had the nerve to say, 'I'm sorry, I just can't do this now, I have to take this day for myself,' because I wouldn't have wanted to hurt their feelings. Not hurting someone else's feelings was uppermost. Taking care of myself is one thing that I do now that I probably couldn't do before.

"I don't think that I measure progress consciously. There are certain things that I have wanted to happen and that haven't yet. And I'm not sure that what I thought was progress really was. My measure is to see what I'm doing and how I'm living my life, the choices I'm making and how they are comfortable for me, as opposed to a choice that I might not have made five years ago, a year ago—those are the ways that I measure progress, but it's only in retrospect. It's not 'I want to be able to do that.' I was never a goal-oriented person to begin with. I don't have any serious expectations except to work on the things that I'm working on and having it get to be wherever it's going to get to be.

"In the last couple of years since I've been going just once a week, I am more comfortable between sessions. I can manage my life a whole lot better without needing to be there to connect.

"I never thought I was an angry person, you know? I didn't think I was a bitter or angry person, nor a jealous person. My mother and I had the best relationship anybody could ever want when I started in therapy. . . I learned a lot about anger. And I learned that I was a lot angrier that I thought, though I still have a huge problem with it. I don't like to go where the anger is. If somebody is really important to me, I'm very careful about the anger. I don't want to lose that person. And I'm also aware now how angry I can get, which I don't think I was ever that conscious of before.

"Being able to think things through better is also part of it. I really never went to college, except for a couple of years here and there and never really learned to study. Whatever I've done, I've done on my own, and I've learned a lot over the years. I used to feel really badly that I never graduated from college. I felt that was a big problem in my life. But I was so terrified of school. I was terrified of learning anything. I didn't think I could! My mother used to always tell me how much smarter she was than I, and that by the time she was in third or fourth grade, she had skipped three times. She never went to college, but she was always letting me know that she was smarter than I was. And so I had very difficult times learning anything. I totally block so that I can't hear what the person is trying to teach me. Now I'm better than I was before, so I'm more comfortable learning things.

"I am much better in my work, and perhaps do this work because I've been in therapy. It gives me confidence. It taught me how to listen. The work I do entails a lot of writing, which I've had actually no training in. I attribute the fact that I can even do it to the learning that takes place in a good therapeutic setting."

Enlarging Our Selves

I could imagine how hard it would be, on the spot, to explain the ways life changed as a result of therapy. I asked the questions anyway, though my participants knew them in advance and knew they would be allowed to amend their comments. But Rose was accustomed to free association, which draws from a deep well whatever, as she puts it, is uppermost in her mind.

In one quiet remark she said she used to make plans after a session as a way of "avoiding dealing with things." We might ask why anyone would go to the trouble and expense of therapy only to find ways to *avoid dealing with things*. In fact we have many ways to avoid whatever we don't want to talk about. We can miss appointments, talk about easier matters, convince our therapist we are fine, or end therapy altogether. Feelings of irritation, anger, and scorn toward our therapist are also useful avoidance techniques, yet all these feelings are freighted with meaning.

We think we can talk about *it*—if we are even yet aware of what *it* is—and then come to see that talking about *it* is too difficult. We think we can work up the courage, but face-to-face find we can't. The see-sawing of avoidance-and-approach is a natural if disconcerting pattern in therapy. If *it* is something you can't talk about, rest assured *it* is one of your issues. Chances are also good that talking about *it* would unlock one of your personal mysteries.

Rose has a long list of betterments from a long process of enlarging her *self.* They include having more confidence, a willingness to take a stand on things, being able to live in a state of not knowing how something will turn out (but being able to remain steadfast), taking care of herself and her own needs, owning all her feelings (she didn't think she was angry, bitter, or jealous), and being able to think things through. When anxiety darts around in our brains, our thinking is more fragmented, dodging from one topic to the next, with sentences incomplete, projects unfinished, and being unable to settle into the matter at hand and focus.

Rose described how hard it used to be that she "never graduated from college" and how hard it was to learn things in school, how she would block out whatever someone tried to teach her. School and learning had been accompanied by terror. As she told me this I looked around at some of the evidence of her many accomplishments. It was apparent that her strength was not based on a certificate bestowed by someone else. Instead, she had looked within herself to find that it had been there all along.

With every obstacle we face and work through in therapy, we gain stamina. This in turn transfers to whatever we confront in the world outside.

NIMH Bipolar Disorder

Bipolar disorder often develops in a person's late teens or early adult years. At least half of all cases start before age 25... Most scientists agree that there is no single cause. Rather, many factors likely act together to produce the illness or increase risk...Bipolar disorder is not easy to spot when it starts. The symptoms may seem like separate problems, not recognized as parts of a larger problem. Some people suffer for years before they are properly diagnosed and treated. Like diabetes or heart disease, bipolar disorder is a long-term illness that must be carefully managed throughout a person's life.[55]

Jenny

Jenny related, "I spend less time feeling like a fake. I used to feel like a fake—and I was!—this false front. But I don't feel good about myself very often. I feel like I'm a good mom, but that's about the only positive thing I can really come up with here about myself. And I know I'm smart. But . . . and I know I'm a good friend. That's three. That's pretty good," she laughs. "That's probably the best we're going to do here. I don't always feel like I'm a good wife. I spend a lot of time feeling that most everybody is better than me.

"I gauge progress in that I am able to speak my truth probably eighty percent of the time now. What I mean is . . . tell the truth. About how I feel about myself, about my history. Where I run into problems is if I'm caught off guard and someone bullies me or overwhelms me, it sometimes takes me a minute to get myself back, to come back from being that little girl and be the adult. That I am able to trust more people than just my therapist—not a lot. It's a pretty small group there. And that I'm able to open up to allow myself to be vulnerable. And it's a pretty recent one in the last few years . . . to allow myself to be vulnerable and be loved . . . It's huge."

I asked Jenny the impossible question I asked everyone: What do you imagine your life might have been like without therapy?

"I would never have had my son. It would have been a tragedy leading up to that, with alcohol, drug abuse, sleeping around looking for love. Self-imploding. And I would have been grateful to have it over with. Before counseling, my life was numb, out of control all the time.

"By going through therapy I know myself on a level and in a way a lot better than most people know themselves. I might still be afraid to act on some of those things, but I know them. I know people who go their whole lives and they don't know themselves. They don't feel fulfilled because they don't know what they need to be fulfilled. I feel like I have a pretty good idea of what I need to be fulfilled. Don't have it yet, but I'm working on it."

Learning to Trust Again

Those who grow up in a family where they are allowed to "speak their truth" may find it hard to imagine what it would have been like not to be allowed to say how you feel—to be angry, afraid, or jealous, even happy—and not have it end in ruin. Those who didn't can hardly imagine what it would have been like to grow up in a family that wasn't dominated by fear, one in which every member of the family lived on a separate island.

Those who grew up in fear must learn that it's now safe to express our feelings, that we no longer have to keep ourselves in check and vigilant. Such learning is like crossing the ocean in a rowboat. It feels that dangerous. Keeping ourselves safe has become so ingrained that we have to practice being nonvigilant for years to reestablish trust and learn that we no longer need to live in a state of hypervigilance.

We practice it with our therapist again and again, trying to relearn that not everyone will explode at us, criticize, reject, punish—whatever the early and repeated lessons were. It is in the relationship with our therapist—that blank canvas onto whom we transfer the impossibly difficult feelings of our past—that we begin to undo it. Over time we begin to relax our vigilance and, little by little, to trust again; it is slow work.

One of the lessons of the experience is to feel that we understand what it is like for people who live in places where cruelty is sanctioned by the parents or the government, where nothing and no one is safe. However, before we can feel empathy for others, we have to secure a relationship with someone that we believe won't hurt us. Until we have that connection to another human being, we can think only of ourselves.

Some parents have the ability to provide materially for a child but not emotionally. This is hard to sort out because it seems as if your needs have been met; superficially they may have been. Perhaps these parents never received as children the nurturing they needed to feel safe in the world. As children, we need to feel cherished if we are to be free to express ourselves and to know what it's like to live in open dialogue with others. For optimum growth and development to unfold families must be able to provide their children with the sense of a comforting, steadfast presence.

The idea of speaking one's truth lingers. To speak the truth of our feelings we first have to know them. Knowing how we feel is the deepest, most everlasting, and powerful outcome of good therapy. When we have a clear line from our heart to our head, the knowledge of our true feelings makes it possible to make good decisions and to live life more fully. Learning how to trust again is not everyone's challenge, but it is for many of us.

Beth

As a therapist herself, Beth works on her own issues with a psychoanalytically oriented clinical social worker. She anticipates a change from once a week to twice-weekly sessions. Being in therapy, she feels, gives her a sensitivity to her patients that she would not otherwise have.

"I have a better understanding of myself, the good and the bad. Being more in touch with who I am is a huge benefit—who I am, how I got to be this way, why I'm this way, and where I want to go. Looking especially at *who I am*, as opposed to where I want to go, which to me sounds a little more solution-focused. I still want to know and digest this—who I am—and understand why it influences me in the present as it does.

"I can carry myself more confidently in situations. I don't know if it would particularly be observable to others, but it is to me. To be able to just move about my life with more clarity of who I am and why I'm doing what I'm doing, and do I want to be doing this—living more in the moment while still thinking about and digesting things on a deeper level.

"When I first started therapy I was in a state of despair about my sleeping problems and anxieties at work and difficulty resolving conflict. Things that I'm working on now in my second therapy are very different. I want a deeper understanding of who I am and what makes me tick regardless of the situation that I'm in.

"Through therapy, I am more able to leave my worries at the door when I go to bed. That also is a cognitive-behavioral piece because my husband will say things like 'Your worries will be there in the morning.' I kind of literally, in my mind, think about 'Okay, before I enter the bedroom, I'm dropping these worries off, and they're right there! I don't have to worry about them now because I'll find them and they'll find me in the morning!' And those things are helpful for me. I guess I'm not as opposed to the cognitive-behavioral piece as maybe I originally alluded to. Maybe there's a time and place for everything."

Knowing Ourselves More Deeply

People turn to therapy for help with troubling problems but with other matters, too, such as knowing themselves in ways they would not otherwise. Beth mentions moving around in her life more easily and having greater clarity about who she is and why. She tends to feel better about herself, not to be so hard on herself, to give herself credit for who she is and what she does.

These may seem like small things—being hard on herself, not giving herself credit—but over a lifetime they are like water wearing away rock. Beth finds herself to be less shy, better able to speak up. In her first therapy she was contending with a difficult work situation, but in this therapy she is working to understand herself more deeply, irrespective of the situation.

In my experience, seeing how we need or want to change isn't enough by itself. Some kinds of change are profoundly resistant. Having someone point out what we need to do may not be enough. While we sort through the reasons for holding stubbornly to old behaviors, we have to be supported by someone till we can hold onto the change by ourselves. Some people can do this more readily than others. Those who grew up under more severe conditions need more support until we gain enough strength to do it alone. This is true whichever kind of therapy we decide is right for us.

Sometimes we don't know how we feel until we talk about it. Talking about our lives in depth with someone can bring about change, clarity, and more confidence. Also, seeing just one issue, as if it's on the table in a quiet room without distractions, and focusing only on that, helps what we learn stick to the walls of our brains. We can revisit the issue in therapy as many times as needed—bringing up doubts and concerns, going away from it for awhile then returning—till it is ours to keep.

Having a deeper knowledge of ourselves lets us be more at ease in the world. The capacity for self-knowledge defines us; the deeper this reservoir, the greater is our strength.

Summing Up

In this chapter we saw that therapy, as it expanded and deepened people's knowledge of themselves, contributed to their ease of being in the world. Among the highlights were becoming more objective about ourselves and others; getting beyond black-and-white thinking, beyond "heroes and villains" into a more nuanced analysis of situations and people; and finding answers that lie within us.

In a good therapy we are supported in our efforts to hold onto changes in ourselves. We learn to work things out in relationships, and if it can't be achieved, to feel more at peace. We learn to find emotional truths within ourselves and to work through issues, a skill that transfers into the world. Therapy can result in finding a way out of depression; becoming more psychologically minded; being able to know and speak one's truth; and understanding ourselves more deeply.

With a careful reading, you also may have noticed other results that were mentioned as ways to gauge and confirm progress. Among them were feeling more relaxed and cheerful; feeling less irritable, angry, or depressed; becoming a good listener; having more courage; learning to live with ambiguity (since life is full of gray areas); being more self-protective and self-caring; finding the courage to make important decisions; becoming more comfortable between sessions and more comfortable in our own skin; being more in touch with anger and expressing it with civility; being more genuine; and having more confidence in the ability to think things through. The list was incomplete, but suggestive. Those closest to us could no doubt add many other observations to the list.

In the next chapter respondents discuss their thoughts and experiences of ending—or continuing—therapy. We see that the journey of self-discovery we undertake in therapy continues throughout our lives.

Chapter VIII

Ending Therapy (or Not)

> ...there is no bright line separating health from illness, distress from disease.
>
> Mental Health: A Report of the Surgeon General[56]

THERAPY is about seeing and understanding. The more removed a family is from healthy, emotionally honest relationships built on a foundation of trust, the harder it is for us, even as adults, to peer into the snowy globe of memory to see what was going on in the family of our childhood. Those early experiences and impressions, beliefs and longings are bound up in our memories. Mere intellect can hardly be expected to sort it out in one reading. Families are different and individuals are wired differently. It can take longer for some of us than for others to see, know, and understand what vexes and eludes us at every turn. Yet that is therapy's goal. With "lessons" and practice we become more adept at recognizing our motives and desires. We see, know and better understand those we love (or try to love), rowing in the waters of our emotional life, deepening our capacity to wonder and learn, to feel pain and joy.

Respondents' comments in this chapter illustrate that there is no defined state of finished, as if someone will apply a seal of approval when we walk through the door for the last time. Rather, a decision to end is individual, relative, and subjective. Ending does not mean finished in the sense of not being able to return nor in having nothing more to say—or see, know, and understand about ourselves. To say you were finished would be like saying, in the words of Winston Churchill, that you had read all the books that mattered.[57]

When we enter therapy we don't realize the many preconceptions we tote with us. Some we learned when we were too young to judge for ourselves whether they were useful and true, or were misconstrued and will need to be unlearned. Children often blame themselves for untoward events in a family. Nonetheless, whatever was misconstrued becomes part of our idea of ourselves and how to get along in the world. Sometimes these ideas cause trouble.

Therapy asks us to look at some of these ideas more objectively to decide if they are worth keeping or need revision. Some of them impair our judgment, bringing unforeseen consequences and landing us somewhere other than where we want to be.

Respondents hint at assorted preconceived ideas of what therapy is and what it can do. Foremost of these, in terms of ending treatment, was how long therapy should last. This idea arose repeatedly, as did the notion that therapy's content is somehow finite: "I've had therapy." These ideas raised several questions in my mind. They implied that there is such a thing as being "finished" and that people will know what finished feels like. They also implied that we can judge someone's mental health by the length of their therapy, as if time could be a measure of whether any of us have achieved our ends in an endeavor such as this.

Therapy that works toward insight, growth, and change calls for a more finely calibrated assessment than simply whether or not one has "had" therapy. A better measure and more durable goal than the length of treatment is whether we achieve certain emotional milestones, get to the crux of our problems, and work through them until they are resolved. How we think about these matters will affect the outcome of our efforts. If we gauge "success" by the length of treatment, then we will try to finish therapy quickly, which is not the point.

I am reminded of the fable of the hare and the tortoise. The hare boasts of running at lightning speed, but it's the slow and steady tortoise who actually wins the race. The hare enjoys an oversized idea of himself more than getting the job done. For any of us therapy is never really finished. If we're lucky (or work at it), we continue to grow, learn, and discover more about ourselves across the lifespan whether we are in therapy or not.

As I reflected on my respondents' comments, I heard reasons why therapy ended and why it continued. My own struggle with these questions influenced me as well. Ending therapy involves specific considerations such as truly understanding what is important to each of us, accepting a process, paying special attention to the relationship with our therapist, becoming independent, and realizing when we are in a better place—at which time we decide if it's enough or we want to do more.

Ending Is Individual

Ending therapy is an individual decision based on qualities that characterize us. Whoever we are, we bring our impatient or contemplative, decisive or hesitant, curious or shy selves into the treatment setting. Therapy may modify some of these qualities, but they will still pretty much describe us.

Also individual to each of us are the issues that bring us to therapy and the ways we adapted to them. Mostly we are unaware of the ways we adapt to situations to save ourselves, to save a relationship, to save our children, or to save face. Sometimes the adaptations we make are defenses. Although they protect us, even overprotect us, they can also interfere with how clearly we see things, how we treat others, and how close we can be to those we love. Enormous amounts of energy are used to maintain defenses—to keep people at a distance, to keep ourselves safe, to keep blame trained on another person, and to keep ourselves from acknowledging painful truths—defenses that often disguise themselves in unlikely ways.

Knowing something about defenses helps us notice them in ourselves and be a little more tolerant when we notice them in others. We might notice that we become a bit defensive in response to one of our therapist's probing questions and ask ourselves, What am I covering here? Why am I backing off? Why did that make me mad? In turn, we might notice a friend's tendency toward a more adamant self-confidence than we believe to be the case; if she were genuinely confident she might be less sure about knowing everything, a little more willing to admit pockets of doubt.

Like onions, some of us have layer on layer of defenses. Finding our way through them to our deepest feelings takes time, effort, and a good therapist who makes us work. Our individual character, in relation to the therapist, helps determine how interested we are in the process, how meaningful we find it, how much value we place on these somewhat ineffable personal achievements, and how much therapy we can reasonably afford.

Someone who was molested as a child feels a burning need to come to terms with what happened, to somehow lay it to rest, while another person prefers to leave the memories undisturbed; these are individual choices and needs.

A range of attitudes toward therapy and emotional life present themselves—from complete indifference at one end to a fascination and sense of empowerment at the other. Where we fall in that range contributes to our degree of willingness to engage in the process. This predisposition, though somewhat malleable, is a strong force.

NIMH Postpartum Depression

The postpartum period is a time of major adjustment for new parents. Biological changes in mothers that occur after childbirth are often accompanied by significant changes in family roles and responsibilities as well...Recently, disorders during the postpartum period have also been described in new fathers... And although psychotherapy has been shown to be effective, getting access to evidence-based treatment can be difficult.[58]

Ending Is Relative

The decision to end therapy is also relative, as opposed to absolute. There is no fixed, universal point for ending treatment. No gong sounds to alert us. A decision to leave is connected to other feelings and issues. Some people will not want to leave treatment before they've explored what they know they have not addressed, whereas others will straightforwardly decide to take a pass on lingering shadows across their lives. We saw in the previous chapter that many people who go into therapy with a specific goal are surprised when they emerge with a great deal more; others are more focused on finding solutions.

One person may know he has not addressed something difficult in his life, but feels "relatively" fine. Another person, perhaps with a similar history, finds he can't live with himself, can't find any peace, until he returns to the source of his sorrow and faces it squarely. There may be no fixed state of emotional perfection that people strive for or reach, but we can achieve relief and peace by degrees.

A decision to end therapy entails a debate between the merits of "feeling better" (and leaving therapy) with "doing more" (and being drawn further into the process). We ask ourselves whether we can tolerate less of the status quo in favor of being open to new ideas about who we are or can become. In this intriguing work we can learn how our ideas about money, manliness, parenthood, sexuality, jealousy, ambition, anger, and love came to be what they are, possibly opening us to a new realm of feeling and awareness. So, what constitutes an end to therapy is relative, depending on how we define it.

Ending Is Subjective

The decision to end therapy is also subjective. Ideally it arises from *within* a person rather than as an external directive. One person's sense of whether any given issue is resolved may differ from another person's, just as one person's idea of money well spent differs from another's. There is no litmus test to tell us when we're done.

For you, perhaps six months of talking about a situation is enough to feel you're back on track, whereas someone else may need a deeper understanding over a longer period of time to come to terms with something. Patients and their respective therapists, like family members, will also see situations differently.

Any of us may differ in our willingness to live with an inability to do things that others seem to do effortlessly. We differ, too, on how much we crave knowing who we are, how we came to be this way, and what we'll put up with. Some of us are more comfortable swimming in ambiguity than are others who want concrete, observable, measurable results. Therapists differ in the ways they assess someone's mental health and well-being, in the ways they relate to us, and in their ability to help clients work through their troubled feelings. "Enough" therapy is a subjective and personal decision. What matters is to know one's own mind.

Sarah

"I would come to a point where I needed to move on to a different therapist to grow more. That's all they could provide me and in every situation we agreed on it. With one, I just needed a break. My last one is still open for me to go back to her. The money thing was starting to bother me. It was getting expensive. So that was the main reason. If the money were not an issue I would have continued with the last therapist, maybe nail it down to once a month."

Struggling with the Expense

Perhaps nowhere is the decision to end therapy more individual, relative, and subjective than in paying for it. Sarah's situation suggests some choices: finding a therapist who is willing to adjust his or her fees, considering a clinic with sliding scale fees, keeping session frequency to an affordable schedule, deciding if the issue really is the monetary cost or something else, and, if possible, finding a way to make therapy a priority in your life and commit to the process.

Christine

On ending therapy in college Christine said, "I realized there was going to be an end point when I went to [my therapist], and we didn't really have too much to talk about. I was doing good in all aspects. I wasn't negative. I had pretty much accomplished what I had set out to accomplish. She had asked me, 'Do you feel like you still need to come here?' and I thought, 'I think I can figure out the rest on my own.' I had discovered why I'm doing what I'm doing, and I'm catching myself. I'm feeling optimistic, and I think I can go from here by myself."

One important lesson was that of resuming therapy when her eating disorder returned. "Lots of people have to go back—it's normal—especially for eating disorders. They stay with you for so long. My therapist told me that she wants to quit the private practice, but she keeps having the same women coming back because bulimia or anorexia has resurfaced. I wish I had known that it was normal for people with eating disorders to relapse and have to go again to counseling. That would have made me feel a lot better the second time I had to go. Now that I've realized it's a common thing, I won't have the same fears I had of failure. If it happens again, I would be very ready to go into counseling to stop it.

"The only thing I would have done different about therapy would be to go sooner. I had the bulimia for a long time. In high school I had it for a year or two before my mom found out. And I had it probably for eight or nine months in college before I went again.

"Realizing how many people have gone to counseling would make me feel better, and I wouldn't have felt like this crazy person who had to go to a psychiatrist. Knowing that some of my peers were going, too, would have made me feel better."

Making the Call

Although Christine felt confident she could get along on her own, she also recognized that symptoms may re-surface. They could be in response to situational stress, or they may signal psychic distress, as some suggest, something she throws up to avoid looking more deeply to understand what is troubling her (those layers like onions). One day she may want to do more work to get to the crux of the problem, or it may have been resolved. For now she felt confident to wrap up her therapy and did so in agreement with her therapist.

Greg

Greg's decision of when to end therapy came relatively easily. "I started feeling better. Sometimes I'd feel fine one week, and think, 'Well, it's time to quit'—but I didn't want to quit too early. So I would go back, and it turns out it was sort of up and down—feeling better, sometimes worse—and it got to a point where I was feeling better more consistently, and I stayed on for at least a few more sessions just to make sure there weren't relapses, and also it seemed like we had pretty much explored . . . maybe we were talking about the same things over again. There weren't new issues after a few months. When I felt better for a period of time, I was satisfied."

Knowing When You're Done

Greg's was not an anguished decision of wondering if he was ready to stop. Such a clear-cut feeling may not be part of everyone's process or make-up, but it was his. He observed that his consistent moods were sufficient evidence that he could now withstand his mother's decline with enough resilience to see it through.

Allen

Allen noted, "I had decided that whatever it's going to take—even if I got to the point where the number of sessions ran past whatever the insurance company had dictated—I was committed to seeing this through." He knew that ending was his choice, ideally by mutual agreement, with the understanding that he could return whenever he felt the need.

Among Allen's lessons was realizing the inseparability of mind and body. "It's one thing that struck me that's different about my thinking now than before therapy. The separation of physical and mental, the fact that you ought to divest yourself of that notion—I wish I would have known that earlier. I wish I would have known that I'm not weak because I need this help. It's actually an act of strength to get busy healing."

He also realized he had tried to run from the problem. Had he known how near at hand relief was, he would have faced therapy sooner. "It had to get so bad for me—and it shouldn't have to be that way.

"Each of us, I'm sure, has different notions of what progress is. You have to give therapy a fair chance to work. It's not a magic bullet that works overnight. To succeed you have to open up to your therapist and talk honestly about those nooks and crannies you don't want to admit to having. But there are benefits that you can't even anticipate ahead of time."

Peering into Nooks and Crannies

Allen was aware of the "nooks and crannies" in his mind where uncomfortable feelings were held and knew he needed to talk about them. The gold seems to lie in the veins of whatever is hard to talk about, then hammering it into an acceptable shape. He had specific discomforts and unsettling symptoms that were somewhat quantifiable, a matter of degree rather than being there or not. He felt that by talking about what he preferred to avoid, he could lessen the impact of a panic attack. And that's what happened.

Nora

Nora said, "At the end I wanted to quit. When I figured out where we were going, and I could see that I was getting there, I said to him [the therapist], 'Well, how many more sessions are we going here?' And he said, 'Do you feel you want to continue or not? I usually go until the person tells me that they don't want to come anymore.' I thought that was fair. It wasn't really complicated. It was just learning the concept, applying it, then coming back and talking about it."

She would consider going again, but perhaps to someone with a different approach. Then she added, "You have to start unwinding a little of that ball before it gets to be huge. You certainly come out with a different perspective and at least will have been able to talk to somebody who will listen, if you don't have anyone."

Having Someone Who Listens

Nora mentions unwinding a little of that ball—of disappointment, depression, frustration, anger, and pain—before it gets to be huge. Talking to someone who will listen and understand brings solace. If you unburdened yourself to someone who didn't understand, the experience would feel entirely different.

Many of my interview participants wished they had not waited so long to go into therapy. Yet people can't be made to go, however obvious a problem may be to others, even to ourselves. It seems that we mostly turn to therapy when all else has failed and we are finally miserable enough. The caution here is that the longer we live with our assorted emotional problems, or doubts about whether things are as they seem, the longer they will take to resolve; the sooner we deal with them, the sooner we can be on firmer ground.

For most of my respondents, once they were relieved of the burden they carried, they were done enough, and that point is highly individual.

NIMH Cost of Mental Disorders to Society

Major mental disorders cost the nation at least $193 billion annually in lost earnings alone...[These are due to lost] earning potential, costs associated with treating coexisting conditions, Social Security payments, homelessness and incarceration...Using data from 4,982 respondents, the researchers calculated the amount of earnings lost in the year prior to the survey among people with serious mental illness (SMI). SMI is a broad category of illnesses that includes mood and anxiety disorders that have seriously impaired a person's ability to function for at least 30 days in the year prior to the survey. It also includes cases of any mental disorder associated with life-threatening suicidal behaviors or repeated acts of violence.[59]

James

"I knew it was time to end when I had resolved—mostly resolved—the issue with Daniel. It didn't feel like quitting. We were done! We talked about it. I was moving and therapy had run its course.

"I didn't feel diminished by going to see a therapist. He helped me feel that way because he had so much integrity in the way he talked about how people who truly care about their health and are honest enough to face things in their lives are healthier people than those who don't. And I would go again. There are things that I could improve in my life. The act of committing to sitting down with someone—even when you don't feel like it sometimes, of being honest and talking—is healthy."

Being Close to Someone

James highlights a quiet side of seeing a therapist: it's healthy. It isn't all about crisis, dysfunction, and illness. When the larger issues have been sifted through, the relationship with our therapist has a different quality.

In *Psychoanalytic Psychotherapy* Nancy McWilliams refers to a "transformative intimacy" in the therapeutic relationship for both therapist and client. She writes, "Recent research in neuroscience reveals that when two people are regularly in sincere emotional connection, their respective brains are slowly changed. As they work out their unique synchronized pattern of relationship, new neural networks are laid down in each party, especially in the areas of imagery, affect, and deep structure specific to the 'right mind,' the brain hemisphere that psychoanalytically savvy researchers . . . have equated with the Freudian unconscious. Our brains literally 'grow' from intimate exposure to the minds of others. "[60]

Of course this happens not only with therapists. Such close attachments tether us to the earth; their absence is noticeable in the lives of those who don't have them. A good therapist can help us revise and rearrange the parts of our make-up that prevent us from having more satisfying, sustaining relationships.

Melanie

When I asked Melanie if she sees an end to therapy, she simply said, "I don't see an end to my therapy at this point, and I don't know how I will know when it is ready to end."

Not Knowing When

It's okay not to know. If we are lucky enough to find a therapist we like working with, and if we feel ourselves making gains, feeling stronger, taking on new challenges because of it—keep going! That's what we want. We don't have to know how we'll know when we're done, but trust that when we're ready, we will. Those who grew up with at least one stable, supportive parent might have difficulty imagining how it would feel not to have something under them as they go about their lives. A therapeutic relationship can provide it until we feel secure enough to go it alone. It's okay.

Claire

Claire recalled reaching a point when she decided to stop. "I was feeling so much better about myself. I understood what had been my problems in the past, why I had acted the way I did in the past, and learned how to change my thinking and my behavior so I didn't repeat the same behaviors. I was feeling much happier, but also impatience—wanting to be out of therapy and not wanting to continue.

"There was some kind of conflict with my therapist because he felt that I needed to continue, and I think I felt at that time, 'Well, maybe after you've been with a therapist all that time maybe they don't want to let you go, or maybe he likes the money I pay him every week,' she said, laughing. 'Maybe you become kind of like a child to them after awhile.

"I wish I had known enough to go into therapy twenty years before I did. I was in my late thirties when I went in. Like everything in life, hindsight is good. I think you have to get to a certain place before you're ready to do therapy, and obviously I didn't come to it until I was ready.

"I'm not very good about articulating my thoughts about therapy. I can articulate very well if we're talking about politics, but therapy was not something that I can articulate well. It was a process, and I couldn't describe what happened, but it happened. And I'm in a better place. I don't know that I have all the words to say how I got better or what went on there. Sometimes I'd have sessions, and I couldn't even remember what happened in the sessions. But I carry it with me. I'll carry the lessons I learned in therapy with me for the rest of my life, and I am very grateful for that."

Being in a Better Place

Like good parents, good therapists foster a patient's growth, development, and independence. They engage with us in the areas an emotionally absent parent did not, encouraging us to explore and express our feelings, to weave them in and out of our relationships and intellectual activities in the outside world, to harness our curiosity and passion to live our lives.

It takes time with a therapist to figure out if that person is attuned to us. But sometimes the therapist is the reason for ending treatment. Something decisive happens that can't be worked out, or we become aware of something that doesn't feel right. It may be legitimate or it may be among our issues. In the course of this developing relationship, we should begin to feel more sure of our choice. It may be the therapist's professionalism, skill, intelligence, and humanity or just his abiding presence. We feel a sense of rapport, or we believe that he cares about us and seems to know what he is doing. Or time and again he has *been there* for us or has figured out with remarkable acuity something that has dogged us for years. We have seen ourselves grow, seen that we can think and feel and do things now that we couldn't before. This is the powerful relationship with another person that brings about the changes we want.

So many factors enter in to a decision of whether to stay or leave, the therapist being only one of them. Yet the quality of that relationship can be a strong determinant. I don't wish to seem as though I am pushing people to stay in therapy, but rather to point out that it is far easier to leave, especially when it appears on the surface that there is nothing more to talk about. The choice to continue is less well known, less well supported in our ideas about therapy, and that is the point for those who want to keep working.

There is a fine line between being sure about a therapist and being secure in the relationship. A therapist can be completely dependable, professional, and sensitive, yet we can still feel insecure. It is possible, over time, to feel secure as well. What we achieve with our therapist translates into the world outside. Maybe feeling securely in a better place is another way to define the point at which to end therapy.

Rose

"We talk about ending, but he [her therapist] says, 'You know, some people just do this all their lives.' Maybe that is the way it will be for me. Maybe it will be once a month. Maybe it will be every other week.

"I used to think therapy would be over in the next three months. If anybody would have asked me in the beginning, 'How much longer do you think it will be?' I'd have said, 'Another three months.' I've been saying another three months forever. The question is on the table a lot now because 'Am I going to stop? Am I going to plan to stop? Am I going to keep going? What am I doing?' It's easier to keep going than it is to stop, because stopping is a whole other thing to deal with when you have this kind of connection to someone. And I do feel that way. That connection to him is very, very powerful. Giving that up and saying, 'Well, I'm going to say good-bye and not see him once a week' . . . I'm not there yet.

"What my therapist says about the time to stop is when it's lost its usefulness. There are times when I walk out the door, and I think, 'I could probably stop now.' And then I come back, and a lot of things are coming up that we need to resolve. So I don't know. He probably will have to retire! One of these days he's not going to want to do this anymore.

"The problems with my ex-husband during our marriage really stimulated all the unconscious problems around losing my dad. And it really wasn't losing my dad that was as important as not having my mother be the kind of mother she needed to be when I lost my dad. Because I really lost both of them, in a certain kind of way, though I never really felt like I had her. He was the nurturing, caring one."

Needing That Connection

A therapeutic relationship of many years, or one that proceeds with indeterminate length, is not about getting help in deciding what color socks to wear. It is about a connection to someone who understands deeply a long struggle to come to terms with something profoundly difficult; it is the connection Rose describes.

Consider what it means to be so attached to someone, to need to be attached in this way, and imagine what has been missing in the lives of so many of us who are long-term clients of therapists, how these lives were affected when the original attachments were weak, broken, unstable, destructive. Consider what an achievement it is, in psychological terms, to be able to form such a connection to someone later in life, to be able to work things out together. And what an irony it is that to be able to be that close to someone is to be free!

I imagine that the sense of self someone acquires from being loved by parents immeasurably, without unhealed rifts or losses, has a different quality that the sense of a self that has been fashioned with a love by proxy, as it were, as an adult in therapy. Perhaps that sense of self is more vulnerable, less hardy and durable, being built on longing rather than on plenty. Yet therapists who do such work give their patients what few parents can. As with any long-term and important relationship, having to say goodbye is hard. Perhaps it happens naturally when we have become independent enough.

Beth

"How will I know when I'm ready to end? I don't know. But at some point—and I'm not ready for that now, I'm not ready for that for awhile—I imagine it will end.

"Probably my one regret was when my first therapist would kind of nod off—I wish I didn't get so wounded by it. I wish I didn't take it so personally. I was angry. I was aghast. But I wish I wouldn't have been so embarrassed by it and could have said, 'What are you doing? What is going on?' I wish I would have had her take some responsibility also. I have no idea what it was, but I assumed all of it on me.

"I wish I had known that therapy is such hard work. I wish I had known that it is based on your experiences with other people, and that your experience with your therapist can take on that flavor—that may have nothing to do with that person—but is based on your impressions and on your past relationships.

"To those who are contemplating therapy I would say, 'Good for you—go for it.' What a wonderful opportunity to have!"

Seeing the Possibilities

Every time I read Beth's last comments I hear the voice of a kind parent who says about therapy, "Good for you—go for it. What a wonderful opportunity to have!" More people need to hear that.

We need to be reminded that what we feel is part of us, neither good nor bad. Whether as children or as adults, we are helped to learn how to manage our feelings appropriately and constructively. Whether these lessons are imparted in kind and helpful ways or in severe or frightening ways, we grow up to accept these feelings as a part of us, or not, by degrees. Whatever the early lessons were—to avoid certain feelings or to be drawn to them—that's what we learn. Somewhere in the constellation of our selves they will find expression, or will need to hide or be expunged. The manner in which they are learned determines how hard they are to unlearn. We need to be reminded that a therapist can help us find and talk about the feelings we tend to disown, helping us to re-claim them.

The phrase "getting in touch with your feelings" is overused, even trivialized, but fitting. We really do "numb" ourselves to keep from feeling (and processing) painful experiences in our lives. They become silent within us, as if the door to a room in our souls has closed. These silences are everywhere, but I found mention of one when I happened on an article by David Hilfiker, a physician who works in Washington, D.C., with homeless men who have AIDS. The article's title drew me in: "When Mental Illness Blocks the Spirit:

Too Often We Assume That a Deep Spirituality Will Free Us from Mental or Emotional Illness. But I've Found That Faith Offers No Easy Cure for Such Struggles."[61] I expected to read about "them"—people who have a mental illness—and was surprised to find he was writing about his own depression.

Because I had drawn the same conclusions about faith in my life, I welcomed his assertions that faith alone can't alter emotional problems and a lack of faith is not the cause. I read with particular interest as he recalled an experience when his young daughter, now grown, gave him a handmade gift one Christmas. He supposed she could see through her father's limited expression of gratitude: "That would have been typical for me: hindered from the positive emotions of the moment, emotionally blocked from the love and togetherness offered me by others. And, not knowing what was going on, I felt constantly guilty about it."[62]

The ideas of being "emotionally blocked" and "not knowing what was going on" led nowhere in the article. Hilfiker writes openly about his depression and the ways it interferes with his relationships with others (and with his spirituality), but any glimpse of his childhood experiences—those that presumably "numbed" him because my own "numbed" me—was absent in this account.

Curious to know what had happened in his early life, I also wanted this man who does so much to alleviate the suffering of others to unearth the sources of his sorrow. Relief from our emotional problems is not a result of how "good" we are, how devoutly we believe, how hard we pray, or how much we help others. Relief comes from deeply knowing ourselves in the company of someone who knows how to read the emotional landscape of our lives and who helps us face what we most fear.

Those who have been given access to feelings from which they were previously blocked know what it's like to have a gust of wind in their sails. At this point they may begin to see the possibilities that therapy offers to those who are fortunate enough to find a good therapist and who have the wherewithal to patiently sift through their feelings and memories until they feel they know themselves well enough to lay old sorrows to rest. It can be done. Some emotional problems and the structure of defenses that protect them can take *years and years* of therapy to work through, even for those of us who pass ourselves off in the world as "normal," which is to say most of us, whether we are in therapy or not.

Summing Up

Along with practical realities, we brought to a decision to end therapy assorted preconceived ideas. This chapter explored a few of them and concluded that the decision is individual, relative, and subjective, overlapping each other like a collage. Among them were qualities that characterized us, which contributed to or detracted from our experience of therapy; the knowledge that there was no fixed and absolute point of being "finished" for anyone; and acceptance that no one else should decide it for us. By listening within ourselves, we determined if we wanted to stop or continue. The decision hinged largely on how well we knew our own minds.

In that collage of feelings and necessities to think about were matters of expense, of deciding how ready we felt to make the call between stopping or going on, and ascertaining whether or not we were "done." Many of the respondents just knew. Others wanted to be sure they had explored relevant nooks and crannies, to anticipate how it would feel to be without someone who would listen as carefully and relate to us as attentively as a good therapist. There was the matter simply of not knowing, and of how we would know. Feeling secure about being in a better place was a reason to leave treatment. For some, the therapists themselves were the reason for leaving. For others, a connection to someone who deeply understood us was profound and not lightly relinquished. Still others continued because they saw, like having an expert coach, the possibilities that a strong therapeutic relationship provided.

An incident occurred in my middle school class some years ago. We were talking about a character in a story who was trying to turn his life around by making changes in himself. We resumed reading when suddenly one of my students brought the discussion to a halt by saying, "Wait a minute—it's not easy to change yourself because I've been *trying*!" Knowing this boy's struggle to get his violent temper under control, I could suddenly see how slowly change is accomplished—not just for my students, but everyone. My privileged perspective also helped me see that those students who had been in counseling were better able, I felt, to put their feelings into words. They seemed to have more of a command of themselves than those students (most of them, including this boy) whose only choice was to act out their rage.

When we are unable to put our feelings into words, everything within us is mute. The pressure builds. Being able to sort out and name our feelings helps us be in control of ourselves and the decisions we make. Our inner world has become more clear, less cloudy.

We are consoled and strengthened when we know our feelings, even ugly, painful ones. By knowing ourselves the past is not erased, but we gain our emotional bearings and can feel we are to some extent in possession of our own lives and destinies. Like the North Star, the knowledge of our deepest feelings—not what we are told we should feel, not what we avoid feeling—serves to guide and protect us.

PART THREE

Concluding Thoughts

The heart has its reasons of which reason knows nothing.
Blaise Pascal

THERAPY helps us know our own muddled hearts. If the muddle were just about a failure of intellect to grasp the situation, a problem in need of a simple set of instructions or a list of rules to live by, well, how much easier would that be? Some of us, when things in our lives go awry, can indeed find a set of rules to live by and make a go of it. Others of us can't do that without relinquishing something vital in ourselves, so some of us go into therapy.

Of those who do, how many find what we are looking for and feel we most need? What ingredients combine to make one individual's experience in therapy helpful, even transformative, and another's disappointing? Why does one person keep working in treatment while another, who feels as much impaired, doesn't give it a chance?

The answers lie in a relationship that begins simply and tentatively by asking questions: "Why is my life unfolding as it is? Why do I have these problems? Why are some people able to have or do in their lives what I cannot?" My memory of the man in the waiting room whose figure moved me many years ago still causes me to wonder whether he stayed in treatment, was forced by circumstances to give it up or, with a shrug, simply gave up.

At that first visit he would have no idea what his life could become. He wouldn't know that if he could see inside his head at that very moment, it would have been little more than peering through a tiny pinhole. Nor would he know that if he stayed and kept working—talking about his feelings and memories, little everyday things that happened, even when nothing seemed to be happening, even if he hated it sometimes and hated himself—his inner life would come more fully into view. The strange, jumbled parts would cohere and he would see the drama of his life in its entirety across a wide stage with all the characters he knows so well. He and his therapist would have peopled that story together, putting flesh on ghostly faces and passion in their hearts. Talking about them would drain them of their power to hurt him. He would have wept over all the things he had once steeled himself against feeling. He would have wanted to quit at least a hundred times, thinking he could do no more, fearing the worst, wanting to retreat from the battle within, convinced the effort and pain were for naught.

But his resolve would strengthen each time he succeeded in doing what at first seemed impossible. He'd go back for more. His pace would quicken once he began to see and feel how far he'd come, hungering for the next session to throw his weight at another closed door in his mind. On they would go, deeper into his story, tying up little pieces that didn't used to make any sense. He would not have believed his own life could be so remarkable, so exciting, so painful and sad, could have such subtle riches. His heart might leap. Not only would his early life be made full and fresh, but his present life would become animated, filled anew with possibilities, and maybe peace.

He would know himself. Simply that.

Therapy starts with a decision to do it. The apparently simple act is part of something larger and more complex that leads to a point of decision. It entails gathering the wherewithal (material and emotional) and sorting out the reasons not to go along with those in favor of it. The reluctance to admit needing help may be balanced by feeling proud to be taking care of ourselves. A concern that our faith is insufficient to overcome certain problems might be offset by determination to figure out the puzzle of ourselves. We take responsibility for our lives and take a step toward the self-knowledge that can be gained only in therapy.

But even the firmest resolve can bump up against a problem in finding a therapist. More than simply finding a name, it becomes a process of locating, interviewing, and evaluating someone before a sense of commitment settles upon us—a period of being tentative. A therapist's insightful comment might be placed on a scale along with the memory of someone we know who speaks comfortably about therapy. Ready access to a good therapist also helps. We might tend to minimize our problems, or not notice someone's subtle but pointed disapproval, and these could be deterrents. An awareness of influences that aid and hinder the search can lead to a more informed, confident choice.

The idea of therapy as a process implies moving forward in stages toward a contemplated end rather than a race to a finish line. This matters. The whole spectrum of feelings are part of the process, including surprising insights, evolving goals, sometimes a massive struggle to face our fears, and a heightened awareness of our bodies' response to emotional stress. In the process we give ourselves over to whatever feelings and concerns arise with a therapist who helps us clarify and come to terms with persistently difficult matters in our lives.

Our ideas about therapy are one thing when we are in its midst and somewhat different when viewed from a distance, with a body of experience to draw on. This complementary perspective occurs later in the process or even years after leaving therapy. One person still struggles with her insecurity in a relationship, saying, "I still can't seem to find that therapist that can really get inside and understand it." Another realized years later that his therapy had likely cleared the way for a new career. Those who have been in a deeper, open-ended therapy have tended to find compensation for their struggle with emotional problems more so than those who left early.

Interview participants highlighted ways in which their relationships were touched or altered by therapy. Questions concerned family and friends, work and faith, whether or not to let others know we are in treatment. A few spoke of the experience when a therapist struck a wrong note. Among their comments were, "It has made me respect myself better, and so people respect me better." "My mother did a lot of damage to me, and I repeatedly sought out similar personalities in…[my] relationships." "When there's no back-and-forth…I'm not willing to tolerate that anymore." "The need to take care of my mother was pervasive in my life." "If only I could forgive myself! I'm still working on that." Another mentioned that "things" can have very different meanings for people, such as a burnt out light bulb or the presence of another person in the waiting room. Therapy brought clarity, changes, and improvements in relationships.

The cost of doing nothing contrasted with the cost of doing something; it addressed issues more broadly than money alone. Hidden costs that can't be quantified may take years and generations to unfold. The traumas of slavery and genocide across a broad historic backdrop are well known examples of events whose effects trickle down insidiously through families. Likewise, the effects of a depressed mother run deep in a child's developing brain and personality, as do the effects of parents who negate rather than affirm their children. Twinges of stigma and feelings of being weak or dependent are also costs associated with doing something about emotional problems. In spite of them, the use of medication to sleep, subdue panic, manage pain, or enjoy socializing can offset discomfort. We tried to imagine our lives without therapy, such as the cost of not knowing details of past experiences in our lives whose memory we avoid. The cost of leaving emotional problems untreated is greater than the cost of doing something about them, even when their "cost" can't be precisely quantified. Perhaps especially then.

Continuing in treatment often meant putting other aspirations temporarily on hold (though not always), and setting aside preconceived ideas and beliefs to be open to learning something new about ourselves. Some people are open to having a coach, risking criticism, facing the unknown, contemplating change. Others are not.

Interview participants gauged progress in treatment, presumably a motivating force in continuing such difficult work, in their individual ways. These included cessation of the need to binge and purge, becoming more aware of negative inner dialogues, noticing improvements in their quality of life such as feeling more optimistic and happy, having a greater understanding of our condition (such as bulimia, panic attacks or PTSD), being more accepting of ourselves, having fewer incidents of panic, handling situations better, experiencing tremendous feelings of release and peace after being able to express extreme grief and anger, being able to let people know when their behavior is unacceptable, recognizing that what we thought was progress may change as we learn more about ourselves, being more comfortable between sessions, being better able to manage our lives without being there to connect, having an increased sense of confidence, stability, and strength; noticing changes in ourselves, such as the ability to learn something new without an overlay of tension and uncertainty; no longer needing to shut down when faced with previously overwhelming conditions; being able to speak one's truth; allowing ourselves to be vulnerable and to be loved. Such changes within ourselves are not binary phenomena—as if you can do them or you can't. They're a matter of degree in developing our capacities and skills.

Among the benefits of therapy they listed being able to handle stress in healthier ways (rather than by indiscriminate sex, bingeing or purging, social withdrawal, or physical illness), having less illness, improved self-confidence and less self-doubt, feeling stronger and less ashamed, having more compassion and being less judgmental toward others, being not so hard on ourselves, finding ourselves thinking in different ways, being better able to deal with conflict in the workplace, no longer having feelings of self-loathing, becoming more "open-minded," paving the way for other family members to go into therapy, having closer friendships, having more energy and being more optimistic, having a healthier lifestyle in terms of diet and exercise, getting more done and having better relationships with the family, being able to live with ourselves, being able to better "understand what's going on" and enjoy people, having greater knowledge "of me" and better communication in relationships, having a clearer sense of identity and autonomy, developing skills to set boundaries for others, having a life of our own instead of needing to devote ourselves to an emotionally needy parent, feelings of wanting to live rather than just exist, having more confidence in our ideas and being able to take a stand on what is important to us, being more empathic, learning to live with ambiguity without quite knowing how things will turn out, believing in ourselves, feeling more authentic and genuine, knowing ourselves on a level that most people don't, knowing what we need to feel fulfilled, being able to trust other people, feeling at peace, and feeling joy; at last.

Thus, once a trusted therapist was found and a strong working relationship became established, the longer people worked in therapy and the more deeply they came to know and understand themselves, the more benefits accrued, well worth the time, effort, and expense. The benefits rippled far beyond that one individual into every relationship in the person's life. If the mother or father was doing better, the whole family dynamic improved. Ultimately, each person had to decide when enough therapy was enough.

Deciding to end is individual. Even though certain personal qualities may be amplified or softened in therapy, whoever we are and whatever qualities we bring to the treatment setting will still define us. Ending is relative as opposed to absolute; no predetermined point for terminating treatment exists for anyone. Ideally it can be explored with other feelings and issues, unless something untoward happens to hasten the ending. The decision is individual and should arise from *within* a person when that point of readiness is achieved.

Studying the Inner Landscape

In learning about others' experiences with depression, anxiety, and other unnamed grievous forces that plague us, I recognize the pain and darkness, the hopelessness, and the longing to believe it has a meaning and that we emerge from it more human, if we emerge from it at all. I am also familiar with the rage and the wish to end it all.

What I don't ever feel is a sense of spiritual community among depressed people or a noble resignation to the awful burdens of emotional disorder. Nor have I been able to find stories of determination and will written by people who struggle hard in therapy to understand what is going on inside themselves, how it all came to be, nor a picture of what they learned. I know of pictures in progress because a handful of people outside of these interviews have shared parts of their therapeutic experiences with me, so I know a lot is going on—all beneath the hard-edged, critical public radar.

If we could see just how many people are benefitting from their efforts in therapy, we might see—not just the depressions and emotional problems and sorrows of lives—but also a detailed rendering of these inner landscapes, stories and pictures of how they came to be who they are, one that can be acquired only in a relationship with a deeply perceptive therapist.

Foremost in the picture would be a portrait of each of the parents and the ways they loved and disciplined each of their children, protected or overprotected them, encouraged or restricted them, favored or punished them, expressed their love or didn't, hurt or forgave them, held them or withheld themselves from them, maintained their connection to them or broke it (once or repeatedly), rejected them or made a place for them, responded to or ignored them, supported or negated them, lauded or humiliated them.

We would want to know how anger and other "negative" emotions were treated and expressed in the family, and the ways in which the person's developing sexuality was supported, or not. Portraits of the parents and grandparents would become part of a mural of the person's life showing crucial events that occurred, because they helped to shape the person's parents. It would also show major decisions in each person's life—what she decided to become, whether he married, and all the details of that relationship, whether children were born, what the relationships were in this family, themes and motifs from the person's original family, how things got worked out between family members and, if not, why not. How did they deal with sorrow? Was the family emotionally silent?

We would want to know everything about the person, and wherever the story faltered, wherever he seemed to pull away from what happened or become uncertain or seem not to want to know, that's where we would train our gaze, waiting to know more. If you said your father had died or your mother had been absent, and you had been in therapy X number of years but seemed to be still without feeling, I would remind you the number of years is immaterial. You must keep trying to return to the feelings around the time of his death, the instances of her absence, because they are there. (How could they not be there?) What happened to you is not just a string of facts on a timeline. It is *all* your story and your mural. By knowing and feeling it, pain and guilt become less severe, delivering you to do and be more of what you want in your life, opening you to new possibilities you thought had been extinguished.

This isn't a mural done with a paint roller but with a small brush such as a porcelain artist might use because deep meaning is found in the small details of someone's life, just as it is in literature and music. Then, from gazing at the picture, you might one day quietly say, "These are the themes and patterns and sorrows of my life. This is who I am."

Before we can feel whole again we have to return to a memory and a part of ourselves to experience it emotionally for perhaps the first time. Our therapist must hold us, metaphorically speaking, while we return to that point of loss, those moments of terror, to the feelings that wait there to be acknowledged. We return to a part of ourselves that was left there years ago. We must return not just once but many, many times, even over a period of years, before we feel at peace, as if after years of wakefulness someone has tucked us in to sleep at last. What we who return to that memory must have is the constancy of our therapist who has accompanied us each time to places of memory we would never have gone alone, someone who knows the way and will support us in facing the past so we can *feel* it and grieve at last.

It might feel as if our dis-ease has fallen from the sky, but our feelings originate within us in response to the world around us: experiences with people important to us and conditions of extreme stress, our feelings supported or derided. We adapt, more or less intact. Our lives move forward; some choices favorable, others not. When chasms open between people, we reach for healthy or unhealthy ways to keep ourselves steady, and may become closed emotionally as a way to protect ourselves. We can live with a rather silent emotional life or commit to a process of knowing ourselves.

With a good therapist, the work can be the most challenging and liberating endeavor of your life.

Notes

1. Christopher J. L. Murray and Alan D. Lopez, *The Global Burden of Disease: A Comprehensive Assessment of Mortality and Disability from Diseases, Injuries, Risk Factors in 1990 and Projected to 2020* (Cambridge, MA: Harvard School of Public Health, 1996), xviii.
2. "Global Cost of Mental Illness" from the National Institute of Mental Health, available at www.nimh.gov.
3. "Mental Illness and Other Illnesses" from the National Institute of Mental Health, available at www.nimh.gov.
4. Leonard Shengold, *Soul Murder: The Effects of Childhood Abuse and Deprivation.* (New York: Ballantine, 1989), 2.
5. "Eating Disorders and Other Illnesses" from the National Institute of Mental Health, available at www.nimh.gov.
6. "People at Risk of Major Depression" from the National Institute of Mental Health, available at www.nimh.gov.
7. "Anxiety Disorders and Depression" from the National Institute of Mental Health, available at www.nimh.gov.
8. EMDR is an eight-phase technique in which the therapist uses a laser point or other object, even a finger, to direct the patient's eye movement in a way that mimics the eye movement of sleep, thereby gaining access to traumatic memories that interfere in the patient's life. The patient, by experiencing these memories, is said to be freed of their power to disrupt. Since the technique is not effective with everyone, the interested reader is urged to research its efficacy in other sources, such as Patricia A. Geller, "Eye Movement Desensitization and Reprocessing (EMDR)," in *The Complete Guide to Mental Health for Women*, ed. Lauren Slater, Jessica Henderson Daniel, and Amy Elizabeth Banks, 322–26 (Boston: Beacon Press, 2003).
9. Nancy McWilliams, *Psychoanalytic Psychotherapy: A Practitioner's Guide* (New York: Guilford Press, 2004), 152–53.
10. "Relationship of Substance Abuse and Mental Disorders" from the National Institute of Mental Health, available at www.nimh.gov.
11. "Depression's Relationship to Other Medical Illnesses" from the National

Institute of Mental Health, available at www.nimh.gov.
12. "Mental Disorders and Adult Role Disability" from the National Institute of Mental Health, available at www.nimh.gov.
13. "Comorbidity of Disorders" from the National Institute of Mental Health, available at www.nimh.gov.
14. "Attention Deficit Hyperactivity Disorder (ADHD)" from the National Institute of Mental Health, available at www.nimh.gov.
15. "The Interaction between HIV/AIDS and Aging" from the National Institute of Mental Health, available at www.nimh.gov.
16. Elizabeth Samet, *Soldier's Heart: Reading Literature through Peace and War at West Point* (New York: Farrar, Straus and Giroux, 2007), 241.
17. Ibid., 214.
18. "Medical Prisoners of War" from the National Institute of Mental Health, available at www.nimh.gov.
19. "Half the Cases of Mental Illness Begin Early" from the National Institute of Mental Health, available at www.nimh.gov.
20. Judith L. Herman, *Trauma and Recovery: The Aftermath of Violence: From Domestic Abuse to Political Terror* (New York: Basic Books, 1992), 181.
21. "Effects of Abuse" from the National Institute of Mental Health, available at www.nimh.gov.
22. "Substance Abuse May Co-Exist with Depression" from the National Institute of Mental Health, available at www.nimh.gov.
23. "Mental Disorders Commonly Start Early in Life" from the National Institute of Mental Health, available at www.nimh.gov.
24. "Mental Disorders in Youth" from the National Institute of Mental Health, available at www.nimh.gov.
25. Andrew Solomon, *The Noonday Demon: An Atlas of Depression* (New York: Scribner, 2001), 364–65.
26. "Agoraphobia" from the National Institute of Mental Health, available at www.nimh.gov.
27. "Mental Illness Exacts Heavy Toll, Beginning in Youth" from the National Institute of Mental Health, available at www.nimh.gov.
28. "Long-Term Effects of Childhood Maltreatment" from the National Institute of Mental Health, available at www.nimh.gov.
29. "Soldiers and Suicide" from the National Institute of Mental Health, available at www.nimh.gov.
30. See Gary Trudeau, "Doonesbury," *Chicago Tribune*, January 25, 2006.
31. "Social Phobias" from the National Institute of Mental Health, available at

www.nimh.gov.

32. "Anxiety Disorders" from the National Institute of Mental Health, available at www.nimh.gov.
33. "Child and Adolescent Depression" from the National Institute of Mental Health, available at www.nimh.gov.
34. McWilliams, *Psychoanalytic Psychotherapy*, 253.
35. Ibid., 65.
36. The epigraph to Chapter VI: Weighing the Costs of Doing Nothing, of Doing Something is from Chapter 1 of "Mental Health: A Report of the Surgeon General," (Washington, DC: U.S. Public Health Service, 1999), at www.surgeongeneral.gov/library/mentalhealth/home.html.
37. Illinois Academy of Family Physicians/Family Practice Education Network, *Maternal Depression and Child Development: Strategies for Primary Care Providers*, http://www.iafp.com/pdfs/MaternalDepression.pdf.
38. "Economic Costs of Mental Illness" from the National Institute of Mental Health, available at www.nimh.gov.
39. "Indirect Costs of Serious Mental Illness" from the National Institute of Mental Health, available at www.nimh.gov.
40. Stanley Greenspan, *The Growth of the Mind and the Endangered Origins of Intelligence* (New York: Addison-Wesley, 1997), 314.
41. "Panic Attacks and Disorders" from the National Institute of Mental Health, available at www.nimh.gov.
42. See Ursula Hegi, *Tearing the Silence: On Being German in America* (New York: Touchstone/Simon and Schuster, 1997), 93–103.
43. Carlos Gebler, *Father and I: A Memoir.* (New York: Marion Boyars, 2001), 227.
44. Vincent J. Felitti et al., "Relationship of Childhood Abuse and Household Dysfunction to Many of the Leading Causes of Death in Adults," *American Journal of Preventive Medicine* (May 1998), www.ajpmonline.org/article/S0749-3797(98)00017-8/fulltext.
45. Ibid.
46. Ibid.
47. Amy Barth, "Child Abuse Leaves Its Mark on Victim's DNA," *Discover*, January/February, 2010, 62.
48. Bruce D. Perry, "The Neurodevelopmental Impact of Violence in Childhood," in *Textbook of Child and Adolescent Forensic Psychiatry*, ed. D. Schetky and E. P. Benedek (Washington, DC: American Psychiatric Press, 2001), 221–38.

49. Ibid.
50. Ibid
51. "Post-Traumatic Stress Disorder and Depression" from the National Institute of Mental Health, available at www.nimh.gov.
52. "Economic Burden of Mental Illnesses" from the National Institute of Mental Health, available at www.nimh.gov.
53. "Response to Trauma" from the National Institute of Mental Health, available at www.nimh.gov
54. Nancy McWilliams, *Psychoanalytic Psychotherapy: A Practitioner's Guide* (New York: Guilford Press, 2004), 43.
55. "Bipolar Disorder" from the National Institute of Mental Health, available at www.nimh.gov.
56. The epigraph to Chapter VIII: Ending Therapy is from Chapter 2 of "Mental Health: A Report of the Surgeon General," (Washington, DC: U.S. Public Health Service, 1999), available at www.surgeongeneral.gov/library/mentalhealth/home.html.
57. Winston Churchill, *On Painting as a Pastime* (Delray Beach, FL: Levenger, 2002).
58. "Postpartum Depression" from the National Institute of Mental Health, available at www.nimh.gov.
59. "Cost of Mental Disorders to Society" from the National Institute of Mental Health, available at www.nimh.gov.
60. Nancy McWilliams, *Psychoanalytic Psychotherapy* (New York: Guilford Press, 2004), 280–81.
61. David Hilfiker, "When Mental Illness Blocks the Spirit: Too Often We Assume That a Deep Spirituality Will Free Us from Mental or Emotional Illness. But I've found that faith Offers No Easy Cure for Such Struggles," http://www.amazon.com/When-mental-illness-blocks-spirit/dp/B0008FARVY/sr=1-7/qid=1170537769/ref=sr_1_7/103-4694570-6566251?ie=UTF8&s=books.
62. Ibid.

Bibliography

Barth, Amy. "Child Abuse Leaves Its Mark on Victim's DNA." *Discover*, January/February, 2010.

Churchill, Winston. *On Painting as a Pastime*. Delray Beach, FL: Levenger, 2002.

Coles, Robert. *Lives of Moral Leadership*. New York: Random House, 2000.

Centers for Disease Control and Prevention. "Adverse Childhood Experiences (ACE)." www.cdc.gov/ace/about.htm.

Felitti, Vincent J., Anda, Robert F., Nordenberg, Dale, et al. "Relationship of Childhood Abuse and Household Dysfunction to Many of the Leading Causes of Death in Adults," *American Journal of Preventive Medicine* (May 1998). www.ajpmonline.org/article/S0749-3797(98)00017-8/fulltext.

Gebler, Carlos. *Father and I: A Memoir*. New York: Marion Boyars, 2001.

Greenspan, Stanley. *The Growth of the Mind and the Endangered Origins of Intelligence*. New York: Addison-Wesley, 1997.

Hegi, Ursula. *Tearing the Silence: On Being German in America*. New York: Touchstone/Simon and Schuster, 1997.

Herman, Judith L. *Trauma and Recovery: The Aftermath of Violence: From Domestic Abuse to Political Terror*. New York: Basic Books, 1992.

Hilfiker, David. "When Mental Illness Blocks the Spirit: Too Often We Assume That a Deep Spirituality Will Free Us from Mental or Emotional Illness. But I've Found That Faith Offers No Easy Cure for Such Struggles." http://www.amazon.com/When-mental-illness-blocks-spirit/dp/B0008FARVY/sr=1-7/qid=1170537769/ref=sr_1_7/103-4694570-6566251?ie=UTF8&s=books.

McWilliams, Nancy. *Psychoanalytic Psychotherapy: A Practitioner's Guide*. New York: Guilford Press, 2004.

Murray, Christopher J. L., and Alan D. Lopez. *The Global Burden of Disease: A Comprehensive Assessment of Mortality and Disability from Diseases, Injuries, Risk Factors in 1990 and Projected to 2020*.Cambridge, MA: Harvard School of Public Health, 1996.

Perry, Bruce D. "The Neurodevelopmental Impact of Violence in Childhood." In *Textbook of Child and Adolescent Forensic Psychiatry*, ed. D. Schetky and E. P. Benedek. Washington, DC: American Psychiatric Press, 2001.

Palombo, Joseph. *Learning Disorders and Disorders of the Self in Children and Adolescents.* New York: W.W. Norton & Company, 2001.

Scharff, Kate. *Therapy Demystified: An Insider's Guide to Getting the Right Help (Without Going Broke).* New York: Avalon Publishing Group, Incorporated, 2004.

Shengold, Leonard. *Soul Murder: The Effects of Chidhood Abuse and Deprivation.* New York: Balantine, 1989.

Solomon, Andrew. *The Noonday Demon: An Atlas of Depression.* New York: Scribner, 2001.

Permissions Acknowledgments

Grateful acknowledgment is made to the following for permission to reprint previously published material:

THE GUILFORD PRESS: Excerpts from *Psychoanalytic Psychotherapy: A Practitioner's Guide* by Nancy McWilliams copyright © 2004. Reprinted with permission of The Guilford Press, New York.

ILLINOIS ACADEMY OF FAMILY PHYSICIANS: Excerpt from literature developed for a program sponsored by the Illinois Academy of Family Physicians/Family Practice Education Network, providing continuing medical education for physicians: *Maternal Depression and Child Development: Strategies for Primary Care Providers*, January 2007, Lisle, Illinois 60532.

Acknowledgments

This book was completed with the participation, in spirit and deed, of many people. I am grateful to all of them for their encouragement. Their warm words of support were like fireflies in the night during the eight years I worked on this book. Among them were Gail Adams, EdD, Carole Arenson, Don R. Catherall, PhD, Carol Haggas, Caroline and Kirk James, Anita Ivy Miller, Julia Rice, Constance Goldberg, MS, LCSW, BCD, Adam Samuelian, Jill Schlindwein, and Linda Solarz.

Others read part or all of the manuscript at one stage or another, boosting my resolve and offering excellent suggestions. These were David Holm, David Hunt, the Reverend Michael Knotek, Barbara Mahany, Kathleen Prucnell, and Phil Whitmarsh.

I especially wish to thank Susan Lipson, LCSW, for the clarity of her insights and recommendations, and Kathy Hotelling, PhD, ABPP, for her early embrace of this project and helpful suggestions.

There were also those whose referral or interest led me to someone who became another piece of the puzzle of how to do this. These were Tony Atkin, LCSW, Arthur S. Blank, MD, the Reverend Steven R. Good, Edmund Moran, and the Reverend Jason Reed.

I am grateful to Allia Cole for being both gentle critic and faithful friend; to Heidi Stevens who brought her enthusiasm and deft touch to the manuscript at a crucial point; to Kathleen Swain whose integrity, editorial insight, and reliability became indispensable. Thank you.

And there were those without whom the ideas embodied here would never have been shaped into a book: Joseph Palombo for his wisdom and generosity, Michael Hoit for his steadfast presence, and those who entrusted their stories to me—thank you. I honor them each of them for their openhearted participation in this project. Without them there would be no book.

Finally, I want to thank my husband, Jack—roof, skylight, and furnace of my house—for his abiding love, throughout and beyond this project, and for all he has brought to my life.

Whether you are named or unnamed, it has been a joy to write this last page and remember each of you. Thank you for accompanying me on this journey.

Terryl Kinnear Shouba